Out of the Darkness

A Bible Study for Men Struggling with Pornography

KEVIN JONES

Fighting to End Pornography and Human Trafficking

ISBN 978-1-63525-535-5 (Paperback)
ISBN 978-1-63525-536-2 (Digital)

Christian Faith Publishing, Inc.
296 Chestnut Street
Meadville, PA 16335
www.christianfaithpublishing.com

Printed in the United States of America

I have made a covenant with my eyes never
to look lustfully upon a woman.
—Job 31:1

Human trafficking is the fastest-growing crime problem in the world. Currently, it is ranked no. 2 and is pushing hard for no. 1. It has surpassed the sale of illegal firearms and is quickly catching up to illegal drugs, which is currently the no. 1 criminal enterprise.

The sale of humans for sex and labor is beginning to be seen by the established criminal enterprise as a "commodity" that can bring more money into the pocket of the trafficker. Why? Because drugs and weapons can be sold by the dealer one time. A human can be sold multiple times, particularly those sold for sex purposes.

And the United States is a prime target country. US citizens are the biggest consumers of pornography, whether it be online, in books and magazines, or on the screen. US citizens have money, and many men (and sometimes women) are willing to pay money for sex. And the disgusting fact that some men (and women) will pay big money for sex with children and underage teens is an opportunity that those involved in human trafficking "can't" turn away from.

One of the primary driving forces that drive human trafficking is pornography. The 72 percent of people who view pornography are men. This must change.

When God created the world, He created man in His image. While man was created first, woman was created to be with man. She wasn't created to be man's servant; rather, she was created to be man's equal. Man is to be the spiritual leader in the home and in the world. Yet since The Fall in the Garden, he has constantly failed in his calling to be that leader. And that calling is not to lead his home by violence, physical and/or mental abuse, or other forms of dominance. That calling is to lead by example, in both his submission to Christ and in his mutual submission in leadership to his wife. He then must, by example, teach other men how to honor and respect all women, but in particular, the woman in that man's life.

Job's Warriors is that opportunity for men to commit to who they are called to be by God. It is the opportunity, starting with the commitment to avoid pornographic and even suggestive materials in which women are depicted as sexual objects. It then progresses to commit men to avoid lustful looks at any woman other than their wife. Finally, it commits men to stand by women in the fights against human trafficking, domestic abuse, and other types of abuse as leaders of the community as they were designed to be.

Job's Warriors teaches men to honor, respect, and love women as children of God, not as objects of desire as the world would have them be seen.

As previously stated, an enabler of the human trafficking industry is the pornography industry.

In April of 2016, Denny Burk wrote an article in *Christianity Culture*. The name of the article is "*The Darkness of Porn and the Hope of the Gospel.*" In this article, Burk found that, "a growing number of young men are convinced that their sexual responses have been sabotaged because their brains were virtually marinated in porn when they were adolescents. Their generation has consumed explicit content in quantities and varieties never before possible, on devices designed to deliver content swiftly and privately, all at an age when their brains were more plastic—more prone to permanent change—than in later life. These young men feel like unwitting guinea pigs in a largely unmonitored decade-long experiment in sexual conditioning."

Sula Skiles, a sex trafficking survivor, ties pornography and human trafficking together, stating that the person whose image that a buyer is perusing is most likely not posing for the image by choice. An unknown survivor has commented that she worked in the pornographic movie industry, acting as if she enjoyed the sex acts in which she participated. She states that her "manager," or pimp, was standing just off camera, with a .45 semi-automatic handgun tucked in his pants. She knew that if she didn't perform well, he would kill her.

There are more stories that abound that show that pornography and human trafficking are intertwined.

Job's Warriors Men's Ministry challenges men to step up and be men of God. So many men are complacent about their roles as Christian men. They accept Christ as their Savior, then do nothing more. But Jesus Christ does not call for a man to be silent, or to do nothing. No, Jesus Christ calls for exactly the opposite. He challenges men to be who they are supposed to be—leaders. Leaders of the Father's world, to stand strong against evil. Jesus tells us in Matthew 28:19–20 to [19]"go, therefore, and make disciples of all nations, baptizing them in the name of the Father and of the Son and of the Holy Spirit, [20]teaching them to observe everything I have commanded you" (HCSB).

But He also warns that it will not be easy. In John 15:18–19, Jesus says to His disciples, [18]"If the world hates you, understand that it hated Me before it hated you. [19]If you were of the world, the world would love you as its own. However, because you are not of the world, but I have chosen you out of it, the world hates you."

Therefore, it easier for a man to just believe and go no further. Following Jesus is not only a daily sacrifice, but it also requires a man to tread in areas that are dangerous and threatening. Many men choose not to take those steps.

Job's Warriors believes that a man who claims Christ has no other option. He must pick up His cross daily and follow the Risen Savior, no matter where it leads. He must stand firm in his role as leader, provider, and protector for those who are oppressed. He must stand by the female of the creation, created in the very image of the living God, and keep her safe. To leer at her through pornographic images, to use her for sexual gratification—either by masturbation or by unmarried sex acts—is not honorable to her, and thus not honorable to God.

Job's Warriors calls for men to stand up and say, "Enough!"

The Plan

Human trafficking is a disease that affects every corner of the world. No place is safe from it. From the smallest bedroom community in America to the huts of tiny villages in third-world countries, human trafficking is prevalent. It touches all phases of life—it does not discriminate based on skin color, gender, age, or socioeconomic status. While it is most known to be widespread in prostitution, awareness is rising of its place in the world of pornography. It is in these areas that Job's Warriors most seeks to attack. It is in these areas that Job's Warriors seeks to minister and to change the heart of man. It is in these areas that Job's Warriors seeks to teach men how to biblically be the leaders that God designed them to be and to honor and respect women as they are to honor and respect God.

The target audience is, in reality, all men. And while Job's Warriors can certainly be a ministry of any local church, its main target audience is men that either don't know Jesus as Lord, or have just become followers of Christ. Obviously, the target audience is men who have had, or currently do have, struggles with viewing pornography, both inside and outside of the church. Job's Warriors seeks to cleanse the hearts of men, leading them to Christ as Savior, and giving them the opportunity to be free through Christ from the sin of pornography. It is the stance of Job's Warriors that if men stop viewing pornography and learn to see women in the image of God as opposed to sexual objects, then human trafficking can be eradicated from the earth, thus restoring the dignity of humanity as it was created to be by Almighty God.

Job's Warriors Men's Ministry

I have made a covenant with my eyes to
never look lustfully upon a woman.
—Job 31:1

Who are Job's Warriors?

- A ministry of men who support the body of Christ (the church).
- They come from many denominations, seeking to serve Christ.
- They seek to step up as men of God, serving their risen Savior, their individual families, their communities, their nation, their world.
- They seek to lead their families as Christ led the Church, leading by example and not by dominance or abuse.
- They seek to minister to each other and to other men, knowing that we are created in God's image.
- They seek to stand firm in God's Word and to denounce images and treatment that lead to the degradation of the women of the world, knowing that they, also, are created in the image of God.

Core Beliefs

- Jesus Christ is the Savior of the world and the only way to God (John 3:16; John 14:6)
- The Holy Trinity—Father, Son, and Holy Spirit (John 14:15–18)
- That marriage is between one man and one woman (Genesis 2:24; Matthew 19:4–5)
- That life begins at conception (Psalm 139:13)
- The Great Commission (Matthew 28:19–20)
- Jesus' Return for the Body of Christ (Mark 13:26; Acts 1:11)
- The Rapture of the Church (1 Thessalonians 4:16–18)
- That Forgiveness is a Must (Matthew 6:14–15)

Mission Statement

To challenge and empower men to be men of God; to enable them to pick up their cross daily and follow the Lord Jesus Christ. To enable them to step up and claim their place in honor of and response to their Creator to make their communities, their nation, and their world a better place. To come together to worship God, to study His Word together, and to pray together. To put Jesus Christ first.

Job's Warriors is a five-step approach to purity and leadership

Step 1 (On your own or in a group)

If you are currently trapped in the world of pornography viewing, then you must complete the Bible study, *Out of the Darkness*, and complete the Job's Warriors healing process as part of this study.

If you are not trapped, then you may move onto step 2.

Find a male accountability partner, someone whom you can trust and that you can confide in. Someone that you can call on, any time, day or night. It's not going to be an easy process. Satan will tempt you. Prayer for you is a must during this battle.

Confide in your pastor or an associate pastor. Let them know the battle you are in and that you seek their prayers.

If you are doing this alone, make contact through the Job's Warriors website, www.jobswarriors.org, and let us know your status. If this is a group effort, your leader will turn in the information to advise you have completed step 1.

At some point during step 1, if you are not currently a member of a church, seek out a church home. Look for a solid, Bible-believing church.

Step 2

Vow not to look at pornographic images of women whether online, in magazines, in books, or movies. Try not to read sexually suggestive books or watch sexually suggestive movies.

Commit to Bible study and prayer at least thirty minutes daily, preferably at the beginning of the day. The important thing, however, is to do it.

Read the book, *Every Man's Battle,* and complete an online questionnaire upon completion.

If in a group, your group can certainly undertake this step together.

Stay in touch with your accountability partner and your pastor.

Step 3

Vow not to look at *any* woman lustfully. Teach yourself, through the power of Christ, to "bounce your eyes." Become aware when you are looking at another woman and learn to move your eyes and thoughts elsewhere. Your thoughts of a sexual nature should only be toward your wife; your eyes should be only for her. If you are single, then you vow to remain celibate until you are married.

Continue your Bible study and prayer. Find other men who are participating in Job's Warriors in your area to study and pray with.

Read the book *Every Man's Marriage* and complete an online questionnaire upon completion.

Step 4

Vow to assist those organizations fighting human trafficking or domestic abuse. Become involved in helping to honor all women and to teach others by example of honoring women. Vow not to take this on alone; connect with other Job's Warriors men in the area and never go this alone. This avoids you setting yourself up for false accusations, or for putting yourself in a situation where temptation may attack. In reality, we at Job's Warriors prefer you commit to fighting human trafficking; however, the important part is to become involved in your church in some capacity, even if it's helping set up for other specialized ministry programs. Remember, the enemy will always be after you. Bible study and prayer is essential both alone, and with other men, hopefully those who are Job's Warriors.

Read the Book *Not a Fan* and complete an online questionnaire upon completion.

If in a group, your group can certainly undertake this step together.

Stay in touch with your accountability partner and your pastor.

Upon completion of step 3, receive a personalized Every Man's Bible at cost + s/h.

Receive a certificate to display your commitment to promote the respect and honor of all women, with your wife being the main commitment.

Continue your Bible study and prayer, both individually and with other Job's Warriors. Attempt to attend an annual time of fellowship with other Job's Warriors.

Step 4 (If desired)

Read the books *Radical* and *Stronger*.

Begin a Job's Warriors Bible study to lead men to disciple men in becoming Job's Warriors.

Receive a plaque and a photo ID denoting you as a leader of Job's Warriors.

To sign a commitment sheet as a leader, and that you will adhere to all the principles set forth by Job's Warriors Men's Ministry, agreeing that this privilege can be revoked if you fall into immoral practices.

Contents

Introduction

Why would a man who is not serving a church as a pastor, who is not a great, well-known leader in the evangelical field, who doesn't have loads of PhD degrees feel the need to write a Bible study to help men discover who they are and especially to help men climb out of the pit of pornography, and to aid in the battle against human trafficking? Why would a man who is fifty-five years old and who has run from the call of God for most of his adult life, and only truly obtained (dare I say, "submitted," for when we surrender to God, we submit to His will, not ours) a relationship with Jesus Christ in 2011 feel experienced enough to write such a study? Note that I said "experienced" and not worthy; none of us are truly worthy enough to even utter any semblance of the goodness of God. Yet in His infinite wisdom and design, He created us to do exactly that—to be men of God who worship their Creator and take on their role in the leadership of the worship of said Creator.

In 2014, my wife, knowing the disastrous effect that porn had played in my life, challenged me to help other men overcome porn. I accepted the challenge, because God often uses those closest to us to help steer us where He needs us. And if you are a married man, it is often the wife who provides that guidance. I accepted the challenge due to my calling to fight human trafficking and learning that pornography is an enabler of human trafficking. Despite what many may believe happened in the Garden of Eden as being the woman's fault (we'll kill that myth of her being at fault in this study), women have historically been as in tune with God, and sometimes more in tune with Him, than most men have been. Think about it for a minute. Who was the majority present at the foot of the Cross? Who responded to the tomb and found it empty? Who believed the Angel of the Lord at the tomb, and later Jesus on the road, when they were spoken to? Who hid the spies of Israel in Jericho? Yes, you're correct if you said "women." We men tend to run when the call of faith is too strong. I know that at many points in my own walk of faith, it has been my wife, Melinda, who has brought me back on track. John Eldridge, in his book *Wild at Heart*, is correct when he says that the male of our species has a desire for adventure and conquest and that these are what God designed man for as men of God. But we men sometimes get that one track mind. Once we are saved through Christ, we get our minds set on what we believe to be our calling from God. It is woman who keeps us grounded. It is woman who applies the brakes and makes us slow down. That is why woman is so important. Do you think for a minute that God didn't know what He was doing when He created her? Of course He knew what He was doing. And that is what this study is about—how to stop reducing women to objects for our satisfaction and to realize who she is in God.

I am thankful for Melinda Lee Ward Jones. We met in a sinful relationship, but Jesus Christ restores. And He has restored us. He has forgiven us. She is my soul mate and my partner. I cannot practice my ministry of helping to end pornography and human trafficking without her. I have mistreated her as a woman, reducing her to an object until I fell on my knees to Jesus and began to learn who she really is. While I am the leader of my family, I lead through mutual submission to her and total submission to Christ. And our marriage is total submission to Jesus Christ as well. God, with the help of Melinda, keeps me grounded and my eyes focused on Him.

But I digress. Let me get back to my point. Why would I attempt this? Even after having a well-known leader in the field of Christianity basically tell me that I was out of line in attempting to do this, that I needed to do this by direction of my pastor; my pastor? Pastors do not call people. God calls people, and He does indeed call the most unlikely of people. For as much as I would love to pastor a church; due to my personal background, I seriously doubt that will ever happen! But I have learned that through my own life experience and by my own act of spitting in the face of God, that I must submit to His desire for me to do what He calls me to do. For I, over the last few years, have finally learned what it is to be a man. And not just a man, but a godly man. Oh, of course, I fall short on most occasions, but now I know what a godly man looks like, and I strive to be that. And I hope, through the grace and guidance of Almighty God, to help you see it as well.

Before we get into the meat of this study, you will need to know a little about me in order to understand where I come from and how I got where I am in my faith. I will share tidbits of this journey as well during the course of the study, as well as tidbits I have heard and learned from others as a result of this journey.

I felt the call to ministry as a young, seventeen-year-old. I had no real church experience. My folks tried to get us in church, but it was an "on again, off again" attendance. I also grew up in a fairly liberal, progressive church, where all was pretty much permissible. I received no guidance from anyone in the church as I set out on this journey. I attended a liberal college affiliated with my denomination where all about God was questioned, it was taught that there were many paths to God, and that God was not the judgmental, awful God of the Bible, but instead a God of love only. I became quite confused. I attempted to do some church ministry, but I didn't understand what I was doing. I said the "sinner's prayer" at nineteen, but I mainly did it to try and fit in with the Evangelicals and because I felt pressured. I was caught between the liberal thought that "God is love and all go to heaven" and the ultra-conservative slant that if you didn't believe Jesus was the only way then you would go to hell. It's not a good place to be caught. There is, I've learned a middle ground. Yes, I believe that Jesus is the only way; but I have learned that it is indeed about love. God loves us so much that He wishes none should perish. He has given us free will to make the choice of believing in Christ or denying Christ. Quite honestly, I found it much easier, over time in college, to just party and not worry about it.

It was also during this time that I became hooked on pornography. I had seen a *Playboy* magazine when I was young, but it never really resonated because it wasn't graphic enough. My first experience that I now know came to shape me sexually for many years, was at around eleven years old, maybe less. My dad, a good man with no bad intentions, took me to see a movie. He had already been to see it and determined that it was okay for me to see. He had no idea at all that what I'd see might have an effect on me. And I can't blame him because it appeared to be innocent enough to a man his age.

For those who remember the original *Walking Tall* movie, you may recall this scene: Buford Pusser is making headway against the bad guys in SW Tennessee who are running drugs, liquor, and gambling. The bad guys think that a certain prostitute who they "own" is the one feeding him the information, so they are trying to make her confess. Pusser and his deputies bust in the door and there lies the girl, naked, facedown on a bed. A man is trying to get information out of her by beating her with a belt, and as he strikes her, she moans. That scene was the first time I truly remember seeing a naked woman. I had always been a "legs man," even at that age, but now I saw what those legs were attached to in all of their nakedness. And I felt the butterflies in my stomach. While her moans were, in fact, moans of pain (according to the script, I'm sure), I heard them as moans of pleasure. I didn't realize that I was turned on by this because I didn't know what "turned on" was. But there is another reason that I believe this affected me in such a manner. My dad was a doctor. He was a man well respected in the community; however, it was my mother who ran the show. Now, don't get me wrong. My mother was not an abusive or disagreeable woman. But she was dominant, and she was so because my dad allowed it. You will see as we go through this study that marriage is an equality thing, that no partner should be dominant over the other, but the father is the one who must lead the family. While there can be success with mom leading the family (and especially single moms), that is not the way God designed it to be. So in this movie, I was seeing a woman who was being submissive, but not in a good way. I think it was God who kept me from becoming some monster after this, for I knew that morally, beating women was wrong. I guess I can chalk that up to my dad too. He was never abusive toward my mother, so I while I learned to be submissive to women, I thankfully didn't learn to be aggressive either!

In college, I was introduced to more graphic pornographic images. But the ones that got my attention the most were the ones in which women were submissive. While I liked porn in which women were submissive to strong men, I particularly liked porn in which women were submissive to other women. What I found that turned me on most was a woman dominated by another woman. A relationship with a girl had recently ended when I came across an issue of *Penthouse* magazine. In that issue was a pictorial of an extremely graphic lesbian scene from the movie *Caligula*. It was too much for me to bear, and I masturbated to the various scenes. (Oh no! You didn't just bring that word into this, did you?! We men *do not* talk about this! Yes, the majority of men masturbate, but it's certainly not something we *talk* about! That's just perverted!) But then, I began to fantasize about women being with other women. And yes, in my fantasies these women were submissive to other women. Travel back with me to the story about *Walking Tall*. If you've seen the movie, then you know that while a man was administering the discipline, the woman who ran the show was overseeing the discipline! Thus, lesbianism, particularly dominant lesbianism, became my own dominant fantasy for many, many years.

After college, I married. I must say here that I was just like my dad. I allowed dominance in my marriage because I didn't want confrontation. I didn't want to make her angry with me. In honesty, our sex life was pretty much nonexistent. Since I wasn't strong enough as a man to ask for sex and I had no idea how to lead, I'd just accept that she didn't want it. So I began to fantasize about other women. And I continued to look at *Penthouse* magazine without letting her know. But I also graduated to more harsh magazines—*Swank, Hustler, Cherie*, etc. I spent a lot of money on pornographic magazines. Then I tried to get her to live out my fantasies with me. She wanted no part in that, so I began to look to other women. Although these other women had no idea about my fantasies, having extramarital affairs gave me a sense of power. I was powerless in my marriage, but with these other women, I had a sense of power and of being desired. Eventually affairs lead to a relationship, which often leads to divorce, so we ended up divorced after ten years of marriage and two children.

I remarried soon after and am still married (twenty-one years) to my wife. My second wife to whom I am still married, like me, had no relationship with Christ, and we basically lived for the moment. While she wouldn't participate actively in my fantasies, she did let me have my fantasies. So for a while, although we loved each other, our sex was often driven by my fantasies. Eventually, that must have gotten old to her. In 2000, she found salvation in Christ. I tried to, but still didn't get it… I didn't get what a man was nor a relationship with Christ was. And I was definitely not the leader of the family that God intended me to be. I was still pushing my fantasies on her, but now she was a Christian and I was doing my best to walk her away from that. Think about it, a practicing Christian is not supposed to be sexually immoral. So I couldn't have her being sexually pure in Christ because I couldn't live out my fantasies. Furthermore, my fantasies would never become reality if she was in Christ! What finally ended the fantasies was her reaction to a tryst I tried to arrange. I believed in my wretched mind that if only she could be put in the situation, she would react in a positive way and enjoy it! This would open a whole new door of lustful pleasure for both us. At least that's the way I saw it. I tried to set up a "date" with a friend of hers. I figured I would fill them with alcohol and then they would end up together at my urging. But my wife cancelled the "date"! And when she accused me of trying to have a sexual liaison with her friend, I came clean and told her that was not the plan at all. My wife told me I was a sick b———d. This cut me to the core, not because she called me that, but because now my shot at my fantasy scene was gone. This ruined everything in my mind. My wife, who as the other women in my life had been, was a dominant personality. And like the others, rather than stand up and claim my manhood, I submitted. So my chance to control her through sex had just gone out the window.

I retreated to my fantasies. But this time, I retreated alone. I took no one with me. I didn't try to live out fantasies any longer with my wife. She had made it clear that she was only doing it for me to fulfill fantasies. She had no desire to participate in the real thing. I had been shot down and landed… hard. She had no idea, and only now does if she's actually reading this! I said at the beginning of this paragraph that I retreated to my fantasies and that I retreated alone. I did, but I didn't. You see, I took my wife with me. She wasn't aware that I did, but I indeed did. I took her deep into darkness. She became the object of my demented affection. Oh, I still loved her madly, but because I couldn't control her, because she wouldn't actively participate with another woman in my fantasies, I took her into that darkness with me. My fantasies became more and more dangerous. And now the scene from *Walking Tall* that had helped mold me became a part of dominating my wife. But remember, not me dominating her; it was other women dominating her. Bring into that the advent of internet pornography and you can imagine the places I was able to go.

I thank God that I never had a desire for child porn or for mutilation or bestiality. But those of you who have stalked Internet porn, well, you know what's available out there. And none of it is healthy. None. These next few sentences, in bold italics to make it easier for you to see, are key: ***The images are always in your mind. You can turn away from the source that provided the images. That's really not that hard once you are saved and transformed by Jesus. But the images are always there. They never go away. And Satan uses them to tempt you, to torture you.*** He wants you to feel guilt and shame. But Jesus is the deliverer, so once you come clean to Him, you must let Him take the guilt and shame. And you must learn to fight the urge to return to the source, and the urge to act on the images that play in your mind. There is a reason that God had Paul tell us to "make every thought captive to the obedience of Christ" (2 Cor. 10:5), and to "pray always" (1 Thess. 5:16–18). For when Jesus is at the forefront of our minds, then Satan can't enter in with the images. It's tough, and you will fail. And that is where grace comes in to the picture. Grace is a gift of God that we truly do not deserve (Eph. 2:8). And while the images never leave, you will find that as you grow in Christ, the images are not as prominent. They become easier to suppress, thanks to Jesus. But beware! Don't let your guard down. You will learn how important daily devotion is to your journey; and if you let that suffer, then Satan finds a way into your turf. You must guard it diligently.

But at this point, I still had not achieved "true" salvation. So a chasm began to develop between my wife and me. And it continued to grow. My wife longed for a man who would lead her, not take control, but take command—take command as a man of God. I wanted no part of that, because to accept that meant I would have to give up the fantasies; I would never have my fantasy come true. Because you see, in spite of the fact that she had made it clear she did not want to actively participate, I still held out hope that she would. Have you, the man reading this, ever been there? Are you possibly still there? Continue to journey with me and free yourself, through the saving grace of God.

In 2011, though, I finally had the saving transformation that I had never before experienced. By that year, we had moved to Hendersonville, Tennessee. Next door to us was a family with which we had become friends. The husband and wife were atheists, and since I was only a Christian in name, we got along splendidly. One night, after the families had eaten dinner at our home together, we got into a discussion. As the neighbor wife began to tell why she so despised the Bible and the Christian people, I found myself defending it. I explained to her the meanings of some of the written Word. She was particularly dismayed by the book of Leviticus, which is an arguing point for almost every atheist or liberal "Christian" I've met in my lifetime. I explained to her the necessity of Leviticus for the Jewish people, and the role it now plays as Christ came to fulfill the law. We talked until after midnight. As they left to return home, she thanked me for my time. She said that while her mind was not changed, she appreciated the fact that I had opened her eyes to a couple of things, but especially that I had talked "to" her and not "at" her. She also said that I was the first person that had not just quoted scripture to her; that we had actually had a discussion.

That was my moment of transformation. I tell people that after they left, I felt a tap on my shoulder. When I turned around, God was standing there. And He asked me, "Are you ready now, boy?" And I answered, "Yes." I fell to my knees and prayed, asking God to forgive me my sins and to accept me into His service. Seminary followed. As I said earlier, I doubt that I'll ever get to pastor a church, but I had to attend seminary as an act of obedience to God. I had to finish what I had never completed earlier in life.

And I guess, based on my life as a porn addict, that this is indeed my ministry. To help others get past it, to help others learn that Christ can rid them of their shame and guilt, that God does love them and wants them to have a relationship with Him. And I sincerely believe that pornography enables human trafficking. Believe it or not, for those of you going through this study, He has something that He needs you to do. And only *you* can do what He is calling you to do.

But first, get healthy in your mind and spirit. God loves you. Walk with me now through a journey of cleansing for your soul.

And as a last note, you will see and hopefully learn biblical scripture throughout this study (who would have a "Bible" study without scripture use, right?). My Bible of choice is the Every Man's Bible, New Living Translation (NLT). Where scripture is used, in most instances it comes from said Bible. If not, the Bible used will be referenced. Most likely, that will be the HCSB (Holman Christian Standard Bible, another translation that I like). If you don't have a Bible, you'll need one. Many like to use phone apps, and that's fine. In reality, though, there is nothing like the feel of a good, heavy Bible in your hands. If you can't afford a Bible, go to our website. We can get you one, at no cost, shipped to you. Most likely, it will be the HCSB. While I like the Every Man's Bible, find one that *you* like. There are many, and they're all good.

You will also need a prayer partner. Many people call this person an accountability partner, one whom you can confide in when times are rough. When you are facing temptation and thinking to yourself that just one peek, or other sexual sin, won't hurt. Someone you can call anytime day or night to talk to and pray with. You may be undertaking this study alone; it is still important that you have someone you can turn to. It may be your pastor, if you have one. It may be a Christian friend who led you to this study. If you are part of a group study, then it may be someone who you meet in the group. You don't need this person right away, but as soon as possible. So go ahead and start praying now as to who God leads you to.

You will also need to plan Bible reading and prayer time outside of this study. This can be difficult, particularly if you've never read much of the Bible. There are plenty of Bible reading plans available. For me, I just read one chapter in the Old Testament and one in the New Testament daily. Many plans are designed to get you through the Bible in one year. Look, it's not a race. But many people get a sense of accomplishment out of the one year thing, and that's okay. The important thing is to start reading God's Word. I started in the Psalms and 1 Peter, but I also had familiarity with the Bible. The key is to not try and read too much. The Bible, in all honesty, can be a difficult read. So pace yourself. And don't forget the prayer part.

I also would like for you to start journaling. I use the date, time, location, scripture readings, and Bible version. I make notes in my journal. Sometimes the notes are short, sometimes long. Sometimes they are faith-oriented, sometimes they are life oriented. I then write *all* of my memory verses. Originally that would be one verse. Then maybe the next week it's that verse, plus the second one.

Start searching for a church, if you don't have one. If you're in a group, it may be the church you're meeting in. If you're doing this alone, you may have to visit churches. Just be sure it is a Bible believing church that knows the Word.

And put on the Armor of God daily. Satan will attack you as you go through this study. The last thing he wants to see you do is be saved, to get closer to God, and to get away from pornography. So expect attacks. It may be temptation everywhere; it may be family problems arise; it may be other attacks. I know you are doing a lot with the study and with Bible reading, journaling, and prayer time outside of the study. But daily read Ephesians 6:10–18.

Visit us at www.jobswarriors.org. You may want to contact us from time to time throughout this study and afterward. That's okay. We're here for you. Everything you tell us is confidential and will not be shared without your approval. You may end up with a wonderful testimony of what Jesus does for you in this journey and want it shared. If so, we'll gladly do it. Anonymously, if you so choose. Or if you don't want anything shared, then it won't be. Heck, you'll even find a section where you can share any testimony you want on the web page.

Now, go get 'em. You got this.

The Ten Commandments

I am the Lord your God, who rescued you from slavery in Egypt,

1. Do not worship any other gods besides me.
2. Do not make idols of any kind.
3. Do not misuse the name of the Lord your God.
4. Remember to observe the Sabbath day by keeping it holy.
5. Honor your father and mother.
6. Do not murder.
7. Do not commit adultery.
8. Do not steal.
9. Do not testify falsely against your neighbor.
10. Do not covet your neighbor's house, wife, servant, animal, or anything your neighbor owns.

—Exodus 20:1–17

Lesson I

An Overview

In the beginning, God created the heavens and the earth.
The earth was formless and empty, and darkness covered
the deep waters. And the Spirit of God was hovering over the
surface of the waters. Then God said, "Let there be light,"
and there was light.
—Genesis 1:1–3

I have read many books regarding the Christian faith, and I have read or participated in a Bible study or two. And in each of those Bible studies or books, each has led with a pertinent scripture. And while this study will also bring in other scripture to show the necessity of God's desired direction for us, "in the beginning" is the best place to start. For as God created the world "in the beginning" and thus caused the start of this journey that we call life, so has your world started from your beginning.

We all started in life the same way. We all started as newborns, helpless in this world that we call home. We were all born in different circumstances, with different skin tones, in different parts of the world. Some of us were born into poverty, some into wealth. Some were born into sickness and disease. Some of us were born the picture of health. Some of us were born to abusive parents, some of us were born to loving and caring parents. Some were born into a life of despair, pain, and suffering. Others were born into the best that life has to offer.

No man is righteous. Romans 3:10 (HCSB) tells us, "As it is written: No one is righteous, no, not even one" and Romans 3:23 (HCSB) says, "For all have sinned and fall short of the glory of God." Every person who has been or will be born into this current world will be born into sin. And there is nothing we can do about the world into which we are born. This current state of sin is a result of The Fall of Man. Genesis 3 describes The Fall. Read Genesis 3 in your Bible.

That Fall is what has put you where you are. While there is nothing you can do about the world of sin into which you were born and, until now, who you have become, there *is* something that you can do that will change your life from here on, and about where you will spend eternity. And that something is to accept Jesus Christ as your Lord and Savior. Jesus tells us in John 3:16, "He gave His one and only Son, so that everyone who believes in Him will not perish but have eternal life," and in John 14:6 "Jesus told him, 'I am the way, the truth, and the life. No one can come to the Father except through me.'" Your salvation is that simple.

God took the sin of man, and used it for His glory.

"In the beginning…" It is imperative that we start here. God created the world from nothing. And He created you from nothing. For if He hadn't created the world, you wouldn't be here, holding this study in your hands, and reading this sentence. God created this world because He desired relationship with each and every human being that has been, is, or will be. And that is why it is imperative that we start, "in the beginning." For when God made the world, He had a plan for the world, and yes, He had a plan for you. His plan included a relationship with you—that first and foremost, you would be His; that you would seek relationship with Him as He seeks relationship with you. And His plan included that you be a man of God, a man to whom He could entrust the care of this world. And in that world that He has entrusted to you includes every living thing that is here with you. And that includes woman. Whether or not you are married, well, it just doesn't matter. God made you, man, in His image. And God made woman from you, but still in His image. And your job as man is to care for, respect, honor, and love woman. If you are married, your job is to remain faithful to your wife in addition to caring for, respecting, honoring, and loving her. If you are single and dating or engaged, it means guarding her purity in addition to respecting and honoring her. If you are single and not dating, it means guarding the purity of women that you meet and may be interested in, in addition to respecting and honoring them.

You see, that is who God designed you to be: Protector. Provider. Respecting. Honoring. You are to protect, respect, and honor the world He gave you and the creatures in it; but particularly you are to do these things for woman. For she is from you, in His image. Let that sink in for a moment. Stop right here, and just think about that. Your first responsibility is to God. Your next responsibility is to woman. God expresses this in Genesis 2:18, "And the Lord God said, 'It is not good for the man to be alone. I will make a companion who will help him.'" So yes, stop and think about who she truly is in the grand scheme of this world. She is your equal in God's eyes, but He wants you to be her leader in that equal partnership. Not her abuser. Not one to be used by you.

So have you had a minute to think about who she is? Good.

Say it in your own words:

the women of my Dreams is kind loving Has a Hunger for the Lord

_____

_____

_____

_____

_____

Excellent.

_____

Uh-oh. Get ready. The gears are shifting with the next thought process. You're going to have your first thoughts of why you're in this study!

And here it is:

Stop and think about that last pornographic image you saw or that last image you had in your mind as you masturbated or had sex with your wife. How about that last woman at work at whom you leered, or the one on the street who you undressed with your eyes.

Is that who God designed you to be? Is that who God designed woman to be for you? An object only for your pleasure? An object for you to use for your sexual gratification? Do you really believe that God created woman from you, to be a tool for you and *not* to be your equal? No. God expects for you to treat woman as you treat Him. And if you treat woman badly, then not only do you dishonor her, but you also dishonor God. Is that who you want to be? If you are participating in this Bible study, then the answer can safely be assumed to be "no, that is not who you want to be."

So let's work on getting that changed.

Are you ready? Awesome! Turn in your Bible and read Psalm 119. Wait! Before you do, be aware that it is a very long Psalm. So in order not to turn you away from Bible study so quickly, narrow it down a bit! Instead of reading the whole thing, just read verses 1 to 40. Whew. That should make it a little easier! But as you read, take your time and let it sink in, and notice the very first verse. The writer uses the word *integrity.*

Okay. Read!

Now that you've read, go back and slowly read verses 9 to 16.

Write the guidelines from 9 to 16 that you found, describing how a young person may remain pure. And don't worry, if you're new to Christ, then you are young in Christ!

Write them one behind the other rather than trying to make a list. Don't worry one bit if you didn't catch each one. That's why you're here. To learn. If you did get them all, then fantastic!

to yearch for it and to Lok the
word in your neart and actshly Do
_it_

Now that you've written them out, you should have gotten at least some of these:

Obey God's Word. Hide God's Word in your heart (that means always have it near to you). Learn God's decrees. Recite his regulations aloud. Rejoice in God's laws. Study His commandments. Reflect in His ways. Delight in His decrees. Remember His Word.

In order to hide His Word in your heart, you must commit to memorization. I had a very hard time with that when I first became a Christian. Quite honestly, I, probably like you, had run into the

Christian (usually a Baptist, of which I am one) who seemed never to answer my questions, but was only able to quote scripture to me. I personally think you need a healthy balance—able to answer questions and witness with normal verbiage, but able to pull scripture to back up your answers. Each session, you will be asked to memorize a scripture.

And here is your first one! It is similar to verse 11.

Joshua 1:8:

Study this Book of Instruction continually. Meditate on it day and night so you will be sure to obey everything written in it. Only then will you prosper and succeed in all you do.

Learn the Word. Think about it always, then you can be obedient to God. Then you will prosper and succeed in your walk with the Almighty. You see, that is another important piece of memorization. If God's Word is in your heart (in your memory), then it is harder for you to sin.

Will you fall short from time to time? Of course you will, so don't beat yourself up. You will learn that many heroes of the Bible have all fallen, but even fallen heroes can be restored through the grace of God.

If you want to learn more about Joshua, read the book of Joshua in the Old Testament (it's the sixth book in the OT). ☺ Joshua was a mighty warrior, but first he was a man of God. Moses brought the Israelites through the forty years of wandering to the edge of the Promised Land. When Moses died, Joshua became their leader. They needed a military leader, which Joshua was, to conquer the Promised Land. But because he was a new leader and was concerned that he couldn't lead like Moses, God gave him the instructions above (your memory verse). And the same holds true for you, even today. Study the Bible. Know the Bible. Dwell on it always. It was Joshua following this direction from God that allowed him to prosper and succeed in the conquering of the Promised Land. Ever heard of the battle of Jericho, where the mighty walls fell? Joshua led that campaign. Study the Bible continually. Meditate on it night and day so that *you* will obey everything written in it. Only then will you prosper and succeed as you walk this journey with God. Read about Joshua sometime. You'll find him interesting.

Write your memory verse here, again.

_____

_____

_____

_____

_____

_____

_____

A quick review:
What does God tell us in John 3:16?

_____

_____

_____

_____

What did Jesus say in John 14:6?

_____

_____

_____

_____

Why do you think it is important to start "in the beginning?"

_____

_____

_____
_____
_____

A prayer to end the lesson:

Father God,

Thank you for all you have done for me, even when I was unaware that you were at work in my life. Father, I have issues with pornography. I ask that you cleanse my heart and mind, and lead me in Your righteous way as I move forward in this study and in life. I dedicate myself to doing Your work from this day on. Teach me to respect and honor women as I move forward.

Thank you God for the grace You have bestowed upon me.

In Jesus's name,

Amen.

Awesome. Lesson 1 is in the books!

You should have already been praying about your prayer (accountability) partner. Make your goal this week that God bring him into your presence so that you can talk and pray together.

Lesson II

You Are a Man

A good man produces good things from his storeroom of good,
and an evil man produces evil things from his storeroom of evil.
—Matthew 12:35 (HCSB)

Let's face it; there is no middle ground. There is good, and there is evil. You are either a good man (a man of God), or you are an evil man. There is no middle ground. If you really push it, there is argument that there can be a "good man" without him being "evil." But what we're getting into here is the thought of how terms are considered Biblically. You see, "evil" concerns, in the Bible, to be "of the world." A good man producing good things from his storeroom, is in Jesus' thought here to be a man of God who produces godly things. Thus, one who produces worldly things is not a good man, but an evil man; for the world is not of God. So yes, you can be a "good man" and not be what the world calls "an evil man (or a bad man)." But you are not seeking here to learn to please the world. You are learning to be men of God; learning to do those things which please God. That's why I say that there is no middle ground. Speaking from the thought of the Bible, if the Word of God says that Jesus is the "way, the truth, and the life. There is no way to the Father except through Me," then to deny God makes one of the world. A man can be "good" by the definition of the world, but if he denies God, then he is not "good" by the definition of God. I hope that makes sense to you.

You, in this journey, are seeking to become a man of God.

Now, knowing what your journey is, you can keep your eyes focused on Christ! And this is also a good time to introduce you to your memory verse for this week. It comes from the book of Psalms, and it has become a huge help to me. When I am on the road and awaken in the middle of the night, I become an easy target for Satan. I am weak, because I am not yet rested, and I am in that "in-between" state. You know what I mean… I'm ready to go back to sleep, but my mind is bombarded with images from my past of viewing porn and practicing sexual fantasies. Here is where Satan tries to tempt me to handle my own needs. For you, he may be tempting you with masturbation, or he may be tempting you to rise and go find a prostitute or go bar hopping in order to satisfy your lustful, "worldly desire." I admit, it's difficult to stand strong sometimes; so you must call on God to deliver you from Satan's hand. Perhaps, over time, you will find a verse that is more suitable for you. Until then, use this one! And hey, what the heck, let this be your memory verse for this week!

Teach me Your ways, O Lord,
That I may live according to Your truths.
Grant me purity of heart,
That I may honor You.
—Psalm 86:11

Write it here:

Teach me your ways, o Lord, That
I My live according to your truths.

Grant me purity of Heart that I may Honor you.

While this lesson is entitled "You Are a Man," the point behind it is to learn what the world (evil) has taught you to be. However, it is necessary to have a memory verse and also to remind you that although we are talking about being a worldly man here, the ultimate goal is to be a godly man. I also suspect that as you go through this lesson, the enemy will be attacking hard, reminding you how much easier it is, in your mind, to just give in and stop fighting. That is a trick of the evil one, the worldly one. So remember to ask God to "teach me Your ways, O Lord, that I may live according to Your truth. Grant me purity of heart, that I may honor You."

It is essential that God is control.

Oh, and by the way, brother… you've got this!

The world teaches manhood differently than the Bible teaches manhood. While there are some similarities, the world takes God's law and perverts it to fit the goals of Satan, which is separation from God. Humanism is a great deception as well, teaching that humanity can conquer and solve all of mankind's problems, suggesting there is no need for God. Now, knowing that, who do you think is responsible for humanism? God? Or Satan? A good friend, a Christian man, I grew up with recently posted this on Facebook. I think it's appropriate here.

"How does the devil keep you from the Word of God? He'll offer you the Word of Man" (Walter Clay Smith).

Identify areas in your life where you have followed the world as opposed to following God.

_____

_____

_____

_____

_____

_____

_____

The sad thing is that when the world is chosen over God, it leads to a whole host of problems. Satan's desire is to pull you from the Lord. And he will use any trick he can to do it. Even when you've attained salvation, Satan will continue to come back and poke around. He knows what entices you, what excites you, what attracts you; and he will use every weapon in his arsenal against you.

Let's look at life in the world: Drug addiction. Alcohol addiction. Pornography addiction. Human Trafficking. Sex addiction. Rampant sex with different (and sometimes multiple) partners. Sex with children. Sex with persons of the same sex. Adultery. Premarital sex. Rape. Robbery. Theft. Murder. Idolatry. Lust. Deception. Anger. Hatred. Brutality. Conquest. Greed. Selfishness. Meanness. Arrogance. Boastfulness.

These are but a few of the actions of a worldly life. You may be able to think of a few more. If you can, write them here. If not, don't worry about it at all. In time, you will most likely be able to add your own.

_____

_____

_____

As I wrote this, I saw a great example of an unbiblical man. I was sitting at the airport in Kansas City. I heard a man speaking loudly and coarsely. I looked up and observed him pacing back and forth talking on his cell phone. It was clear that he was agitated. He was talking about someone with whom he worked. As he continued to get agitated, he said to the other party, "I can tell you this, he will fail. I can tell you, he will fail." It was clear that he wanted to see another man fail.

So now I ask you this question: "Were his actions of a godly man, or those of a worldly man?" Does a godly man want to see people fail or to succeed? Or let's ask this another way. "Does a godly man want to see another man (or woman) miss salvation in Christ and thus spend eternity in hell? So, based on this, do you think this man I witnessed behaving so badly has even given his own eternity a thought? I seriously doubt it. Whether or not he is a church goer, I can't say. But I can say that the world controls him. His actions leave no doubt about that.

Dictionary.com defines manhood as the following: "the state or time of being a man or adult male person; male maturity; traditional manly qualities; maleness, as distinguished from femaleness; virility, potency; male genitalia; men collectively; the state of being human."

Interesting. Nothing at all in these words that really describe what a man is, or who he is supposed to be. In the eyes of the world, a good man is one who treats people nicely. I would say that he also works hard, but in our modern world, even that is not required to be "good."

So it's no wonder that men are lost. It's no wonder that men can't find their way. Men have no idea who they are. God wants men to be leaders of their families and of the creation. Satan has certainly succeeded in taking away a man's identity.

Who Am I?

In addition to such a miniscule definition of manhood, let's not forget the fact of the feminization of men! The world (evil) wants to see men not be men! Being a man, an adventurer, a conqueror is now frowned upon! Opening a door for a lady, letting a lady go first, is now seen as a man trying to be the superior sex, and he is often accused of being against women's rights! He is considered a chauvinist!

How does a man know who he is supposed to be in our modern times? It seems that any way that he turns, any road that he takes, he will be maligned for doing so.

Where, oh where, is man to turn?

Is he supposed to be Rambo? Braddock? Bond? Shaft? Super Fly? Solo? Skywalker? Suave, debonair, strong men all. Is that the normal male? I've never understood how those guys can have so many adversaries and defeat them all, whether in hand to hand combat, knife fights, or gun fights. They never lose! I am even more amazed how they escape a hail of bullets (or laser beams) without a scratch while they mow down dozens of the men shooting at them! It is fantasy. And not the normal man's life; the one who is trying his best to keep his own head above water while trying to keep his family afloat or, even worse, trying to keep his family (or society if he doesn't have a family) unaware of his life trapped in pornography or having sex with prostitutes, or visiting strip clubs, both of which have a high number of human trafficking victims in their "dens."

Ouch! Wasn't expecting that last one, were ya?! I kind of just threw that one in on you. Low shot, huh? Well, it really wasn't meant to be. Because it's who many men are. I never used prostitutes, and believe it or not, I've never been to a strip club (I know, some of you are thinking, "liar"; but it's true. I never have). But I have been a huge user of pornographic material and I have watched countless pornographic movies prior to my salvation in Christ.

Enough of that! Let's move on, but before moving forward, let's do a quick review.

What do you think is your biggest worldly (sinful) issue?

Lying and Porn

Okay. Now, list two or three more that you know are an issue for you.

1. _Porn_
2. _Lying_
3. _coning_

Based on these answers, is it your desire to honor yourself, or to honor God?

Honor God

Finally, what definition of manhood above most fits your viewpoint currently? _____

Write this week's memory verse here:

_____

_____

_____

_____

———————————————————————

———————————————————————

Excellent!

Now, move forward and begin your journey home.

Ending Prayer

Father, I am discovering that I have been a man of the world, a man who has gone against what You want for me, and, also, for Your creation. Lord, as I move forward, help me to become the man that You want me to be.

In Christ's name, amen.

All right! Lesson 2 is done!

Don't forget to talk and pray with your prayer partner.

Ask God to reveal to you what it is that makes you tick with porn. What attracts you to it? Not only that, but what triggered it? Remember, for me it became a power issue. It is not just the images that draw you; they keep you locked in. Something caused this. Once God has revealed it, begin praying to Him to remove it. It is of Satan. Something he uses to control you and separate you from God. You may have to call out the sin issue by name, through your relationship with Jesus to remove it.

Take a look at the book *The Bondage Breaker* by Neal Anderson. It's a great help in identifying and calling out attacks by the enemy.

Press on!

Lesson III

You Are a Man of God

[11]Put on all of God's armor so that you will be able to stand firm against all strategies and tricks of the Devil. [12]For we are not fighting against people made of flesh and blood, but against the evil rulers and authorities of the unseen world, against those mighty powers of darkness who rule this world, and against wicked spirits in the heavenly realms. [13]Use every piece of God's armor to resist the enemy in the time of evil, so that after the battle you will still be standing firm. [14]Stand your ground putting on the sturdy belt of truth and the body armor of God's righteousness. [15]For shoes, put on the peace that comes from the Good News, so that you will be full prepared. [16]In every battle you will need faith as our shield to stop the fiery arrows aimed at you by Satan. [17]Put on salvation as your helmet, and take the sword of the Spirit, which is the word of God. [18]Pray at all times and on every occasion in the power of the Holy Spirit. Stay alert and be persistent in your prayers for Christians everywhere.

—Ephesians 6:11–18

And so, your journey truly begins here. And this journey will be a battle. I recommend that every morning, during your prayer time, that you put on the armor of God. You will need it. You are traversing into the land of the enemy. In reality, if you are participating in this Bible study, then you have been in that land for an amount of time, and you were "of the world." The difference now? You are a threat to evil, to Satan. When you were of the world, you were no threat. But now you are. So prepare yourself by putting on the armor. Daily. What Paul is addressing in the passage above is spiritual warfare. Believe it or not, there are forces unseen that influence all people.

There is one other thing that you need to do before you move into the next section. You need to familiarize yourself with the Ten Commandments as listed in the front of this section. These Ten Commandments given by God are the essence of who a man of God is.

Write them below:

1. _____
2. _____
3. _____
4. _____
5. _____
6. _____
7. _____
8. _____
9. _____
10. _____

Honor these, and you honor God. ☺

In this lesson, you are learning that you are a man of God. This lesson will be the most extensive one in this study. It may be wise, if you are doing this study on a week to week basis, that you divide this into two weeks. There's going to be a lot, and I mean *a lot* of information.

Let's start with The Flood—after the ark lands and Noah and his family leave the ark. Here is what God said to Noah:

"¹God blessed Noah and his sons and said to them, "Be fruitful and multiply and fill the earth. ²The fear and terror of you will be in every living creature on the earth, every bird of the sky, every creature that crawls on the ground, and all the fish of the sea. They are placed under your authority. ³Every living creature will be food for you; as I gave the green plants, I have given you everything. ⁴However, you must not eat meat with its lifeblood in it. ⁵I will require the life of every animal and every man for your life and your blood. I will require the life of each man's brother for a man's life. ⁶Whoever sheds man's blood, his blood will be shed by man, for God made man in His image" (Genesis 9:1–6, HCSB).

There are several points in this passage. Hopefully, you have already seen them. First, notice that God tells Noah and his sons that every creature on the earth will fear humanity. Think about that. Unless you are threatening a wild animal's young, the majority of the time a creature will flee from you. Why? Because *they* know the hierarchy of the creation! They know that you are created in the very image of God, and they are not. But also remember that they are in your care. To abuse an animal is to disrespect the order of creation and your position as caretaker! Yet God also here gives permission to eat meat. Prior to the Flood, man ate vegetation. But also notice that God shows the importance of human life. He says that any animal or any man that kills man will lose their own life. Now, in our world, we have courts to find justice, so it is not your place or my place to seek justice through vengeance or by killing another because we know they are "guilty." So don't think I'm saying that! I'm simply pointing out how important you, and every other human being is, to God. If you are made in His image, then that means every other man is also made in His image. Ahhh, but so is every woman. Makes this whole thing of living for yourself and for your own pleasure kind of selfish, doesn't it? You see, God loves you. And he loves all men. And all women. What He is saying here is that each of us is so important, that if harm comes to any of us by any means, then serious consequences follow. In other words, love each other, as He loves us. That's really pretty simple.

If you haven't had a lot of Bible teaching in the past, here's a quick recap on The Flood. After The Fall (lesson 1), humanity flourished, but it also became more and more evil, influenced by Satan rather than God. Eventually, God became disgusted with it and decided to end human life. Yet He found that Noah was a righteous man, so He instructed Noah to build the ark and to take his family inside with him, along with 2 (male and female) of every living creature. God then flooded the earth and drowned all of the rest of humanity and creatures. So, what you've read above was the start of all anew.

God took the sin of man and used it for His glory.

However, it is obvious that as humanity once again began to multiply, we began to once again screw it all up! Yet with this quick story, and God creating *you* to be a man of God, I have had you start your journey after Noah leaves the ark. While we won't be able to go through the whole Bible in this study, we will indeed hit the highs and lows of various people who have faced struggles, some similar to yours, in their quest to be men of God.

Discuss what you learned about man's call to humanity and the earth from the above reading in this study.

_____

_____

_____

_____

_____

_____

_____

_____

_____

_____

_____

_____

_____

_____

Respecting God's creation, but not worshipping it, is worthy.

_____

Let's next look at Abraham. Read in your Bible his story. It is a rather long read, but you need to be familiar with him. For the highlights, read Genesis 12, 15, 16, 17:1–8 and 15–27; 18:1–15, 21:1–21, 22. Be aware that Abraham was first called Abram until God changed his name to Abraham.

Abraham, or Abram, as he is called early on, is the founder, through God, of who you are. Wait. I thought *Adam* was. Well, yes. He was. As was Noah. Whew. This gets kind of confusing! But you see, Abram was through whom God founded the nation of Israel. Abram, who became Abraham, fathered Isaac. Isaac fathered Jacob. And God changed Jacob's name from Jacob to Israel! Sometimes you'll hear the nation of Israel referred to as the nation of Jacob. Anyway,

Abraham is the father of the nation of Israel. Because God promised Abraham that if he would but follow God's call, this would be so. And you'll also learn that Jesus came through the line of the nation of Israel. Hmmm, interesting. And it was Jesus's saving grace that was extended to the Gentiles...... of which you and I are! Oh, heck. We'll get to all of that! Let's talk about Abram—er, ah, Abraham!

I'll try to do a quick recap of what you've read. In Genesis 12, you read that Abram was called by God to leave his country and go to the land that God would show him. But think about that—God not only called him to leave his country, but also to leave everything and everyone that he knew! God also tells Abram that he will make him a "great nation." What was Abram's response? Did he hesitate like you or I do? No. The scripture says that he departed as the Lord instructed him. It was that simple. God called. Abram responded. Kind of like he is calling you now. ☺

If you are participating in this Bible study, then you have a pornography problem. God may be calling you right now to put those things aside and to depend on Him. What do you think, right now, without going too deep, that God is calling *you* to do? _____

_____

_____

_____

_____

_____

_____

Based on God's call to Abram, he must have been a righteous man. However, notice what he did at the end of Genesis 12. Abram so feared the Egyptians that he told Pharoah that Sarai (later called Sarah) was not his wife, but instead was his sister. Not very manly, is it? He showed no honor to his wife at all, letting the Egyptian king have sex with his wife to spare his own life. And as you see, the

Egyptian king was not happy about it, because it brought trouble from God upon him. What I want you to see here is this: we often feel that we're not worthy to be loved by God or to serve Him. Take heart, brother. Abram gave away *his wife*, yet God fathered a nation through him and blessed him.

In Genesis 15, God makes His covenant with Abram concerning his future heir. What is it that God promises Abram? _____

_____

_____

_____

_____

_____

_____

_____

_____

In Genesis 16, you learn that both Abram and Sarai lose patience with God, and Sarai tells Abram to have sex with her servant, Hagar. Hagar births Abram a son, Ishmael. This saga leads into the following chapters of Genesis, as God once again, in 17, tells Abram that He will bless him with a son. He also changes Abram's name to Abraham, and Sarai's to Sarah. But when God tells Abraham he will be blessed with a son, Abraham laughs at him.

What you're seeing is Abraham, who so obediently picked up and moved as directed by God, became unsure of God's plan. How could he, an old man, and Sarah, an old woman, have a son? He and Sarah went outside of God's plan and produced a son through a servant. In ancient Israel, the firstborn son was a big deal. All things passed through the male, so the firstborn son inherited the name and wealth of the father. It was crucial that Abraham obey. Because he didn't, he set forth a series of events that shake the earth even today. Hmmmm… even Adam seemed to have a problem with that, didn't he? Disobedience led to his expulsion from the Garden!

However, God, as you found out, did deliver. He delivered Isaac to Abraham and Sarah. He delivered the nation of Israel through Isaac. Originally, God told Abraham He would make Abraham the father of a great nation. But due to Abraham's disobedience, God instead told him that He would make Abraham the father of not just one nation, but of a multitude of nations (Genesis 17:4). This, brother, is significant. God didn't *punish* Abraham; rather, Abraham's impatience with God (leading to disobedience) caused a calamity of events! You see, Ishmael, the son produced by Hagar, was the father of the Arab nations! See what disobedience set forth?! A conflict that continues even to this day! You may not have realized that the births of Ishmael and Isaac, due to Abraham and Sarah's disobedience, set into motion a conflict that is thousands of years old.

Obedience to God is vital, as seen in the final bit of discussion on Abraham. Abraham finally learned how important obedience is, as he followed God's final test to offer his son as a sacrifice. This really flies in the face of how God instructed His people to worship Him. Human sacrifice was not allowed in worship of God, as many pagan religions practiced such awful sacrifices. So this was an ultimate test (and no, it is not okay to sacrifice someone. If you ever feel you're supposed to do that, you are 100 percent wrong. I only say that because this study is designed for newly restored Christians who have come from rougher lifestyles than the average "middle class" church-goer!). The importance of this last action is to show that Abraham obeyed. But what happened? In the end, God rewarded Abraham's obedience by providing him a ram for sacrifice instead.

God took the sin of man, and used it for His glory.

This is significant as to who you are in God. Later in this study, you will learn why. So bear with it!

Take a few moments here and think about how disobedience may have gotten you to the point that you now find yourself. But don't do it alone. Here, try this: *Father God. I know I have been a sinful man, but as you showed patience with Abraham, I, too, know you show patience with me. I ask for Your guidance here, Lord. Reveal to me my disobedience, O God. And then reveal to me how to rid myself of that disobedience and begin a life of obedience to You.*

Record here what the Lord has revealed to you, both disobedience and how you can let Him lead you to obedience.

_____

_____

_____

_____

_____

_____

_____

_____

_____

_____

_____

_____

_____

_____

_____

_____

_____

_____

Before we move on, this may be a great place to break for this week! So, let's end it with your memory verse, and we'll use this one for this week and next week! (Oops—this one is a little long).

⁷Keep asking, and it will be given to you. Keep searching, and you will find. Keep knocking, and the door will be opened to you. ⁸For everyone who asks receives, and the one who searches finds, and to the one who knocks, the door will be opened. (Matthew 7:7–8, HCSB)

Write your memory verse here:

_____

_____

_____

_____

_____

_____

_____

_____

The next man we want to check out is David. If you have any knowledge whatsoever of the Bible, you have heard the story of David and Goliath. And that is indeed the David that you are going to learn about. Because there is more to David that his killing a giant—much, much more. There will be only a few areas highlighted, but you may want to delve deeper into his story. It is told in the Old Testament Books of 1 and 2 Samuel and the first two chapters of 1 Kings. Many of the Psalms are attributed to David; in fact, when you check out Psalms, you'll see that many are called "A Davidic Psalm," meaning it is believed to have been written by him or about him.

David is an interesting character, as you will learn. Samuel was the prophet that was trusted by David and also Saul, the king before David. In fact, Saul so feared David that he sought to have David killed. David actually had the opportunity to instead kill Saul, but he spared his life. That is a godly man who made a godly decision. Yet

David, "a man after God's own heart," (1 Samuel 13:14, Acts 13:22) was far, far from perfect. He was, after all, only a man.

David anointed as King by Samuel.

In 1 Samuel 8, God tells the prophet Samuel to fulfill Israel's wish and give them a king, against God's will. Saul is appointed king, but Saul fails to follow God's instructions and falls out of favor with God, allowing for the rise of David as king. David is a bedrock of faith in God, which shows in his confrontation with Goliath, the giant of the Philistines (I'm assuming that most are familiar with this story. If not, check out 1 Samuel 17, it'll get you what you need).

David replaces Saul as king, and David is blessed by God beyond measure. But as with the case with all of us in the human race, it's just not enough. It doesn't take long before David screws it all up! Israel, at the time David became king, was divided—Israel to the north and Judah to the south. David united the kingdoms as one. God blessed David with great treasure, unity, and conquests. David moved the Ark of the Covenant, which contained the tablets of the Ten Commandments, to Jerusalem. By now, the prophet Samuel has died and Nathan is the prophet trusted by David.

In 2 Samuel 7 God, through Nathan, delivers a message to David. What was that message?

_____

_____

_____

_____

_____

_____

_____

_____

_____

_____

_____

_____

_____

_____

_____

_____

_____

But daggone it, it just seems that no matter what God blesses us with, we just seem to do something stupid. And so it was with David. Here was a man greatly blessed with a kingdom and great riches. People respected him and bowed to him in service. Men across the known world feared his name. But, he, like many of us men, just couldn't keep it in his pants. Enter into the picture a woman by the name of Bathsheba. Ugh!

If you are not familiar with this story, then get ready! You are going to find that if God extended grace to David after all he did and took David's screwup and made it into something amazing, then you will see that God can certainly extend grace to you and take you on a journey as well. He may not use you in the way he used David, but he can certainly use you to reach people that others can't reach. I mean, here I am sitting here writing a Bible study on how to get away from porn!

You can find the story of David and Bathsheba in 2 Samuel 11:1–12:12. Read the story.

Interesting, huh? Now, summarize it here (oh, I'm giving you plenty of space on this one!).

_____

_____

_____

_____

_____
_____
_____
_____
_____
_____
_____
_____
_____
_____
_____
_____
_____
_____
_____
_____
_____
_____
_____
_____
_____
_____
_____
_____
_____
_____
_____
_____
_____
_____

What was the result? Read 2 Samuel 12:13–25 and summarize here:

_____
_____
_____

_____

_____

_____

_____

_____

_____

_____

_____

_____

_____

_____

_____

_____

_____

_____

_____

Wow. How about that. King David. A man after God's own heart. A man so blessed by God. Yet here he is. A peeping Tom. An adulterer. A liar. A conniver. (Remember, he gave the man he was having killed the very letter to deliver that brought his death), a murderer. And although he was punished greatly by God, he was also forgiven his sins.

As you read, once Uriah, Bathsheba's husband, was killed and Bathsheba had mourned, David brought her to the palace and married her. Don't forget that she was pregnant, which was the reason that David tried to get Uriah to sleep with her while home from battle. He was trying to cover up his immorality. Of course, you know what happened from there—when that didn't work, David had him killed. As you saw, the son they had was taken by God. Yet they were blessed later with a son whom they named Solomon. Solomon is the one who succeeds David, and is the one whom God instructs to build the temple.

God took the sin of man and used it for His glory.

You will learn more about David and Bathsheba later in this study. Be ready. ☺

While there are many, many prominent figures in the Bible, and all but one who struggled with godliness vs. worldliness (humanness), there is only one more to bring forth in this section of you as a godly man.

———————————————————————————————

————————————

And he is the Apostle Paul.

You may not be aware, but the majority of the New Testament contains letters and writings of this man. Writings credited to Paul include Romans, 1 and 2 Corinthians, Galatians, Ephesians, Philippians, Colossians, 1 and 2 Thessalonians, 1 and 2 Timothy, Titus, and Philemon.

Paul was also the first Christian missionary, as he travelled from town to town throughout the Roman empire bringing the Good News (Gospel) of Jesus Christ to Jews and Gentiles (you and me) alike.

I hear many speak of having a "radical salvation." Paul definitely had a radical salvation. In fact, it's probably one of *the* most radical, if not the most. Our individual salvation experiences are all radical, because it takes a radical act by God to extend His grace to us. And when it really comes down to it, when we come to know Jesus truly, we each go through a radical transformation. So I don't personally believe that anyone's salvation is any more radical or any better than anyone else's. I think that when we claim that, we put ourselves above others. We somehow elevate ourselves to a special status with God. And I think that is dangerous ground.

That being said there are some of us that are more deeply mired in sin than others. And some of us are just downright meaner than others prior to our salvation. I believe that Paul fits that last sentence prior to his own salvation.

Paul was originally known as Saul (not to be confused with King Saul of David's time). He was not a good man. Saul was a devout Jew who followed the Jewish law. He had no time for these new Christian folk, these followers of Jesus. The first mention of Saul in the Bible is in the book of Acts. The book of Acts describes the life of the early church and the actions of the disciples of Jesus after His ascension to heaven following His resurrection. Saul's first acknowledgment is in Acts 7:57–8:1. It involves the death of a new disciple of Jesus, Stephen:

[57] Then they put their hands over their ears and began shouting. They rushed at him and dragged him out of the city [58] and began to stone him. His accusers took off their coats and laid them at the feet of a young man named Saul. [59] As they stoned him, Stephen prayed, "Lord Jesus, receive my spirit." [60] He fell to his knees, shouting, "Lord, don't charge them with this sin!"

[1] And with that, he died. Saul was one of the witnesses, and he agreed completely with the killing of Stephen.

Wow. This is important in scripture. You see, Saul was not considered, even by the world's standards, to be a good man. He was a terrible persecutor of the new Christian movement, referred to then as "The Way." He was just bad news. He literally went from door to door searching for people of "The Way" in order to destroy them. The Bible doesn't record how many Christian deaths he may have had a hand in, if any, but even Paul, in Acts 22:19–20, said this:

[19] "But Lord," I argued, "they certainly know that in every synagogue I imprisoned and beat those who believed in you. [20] And I was in complete agreement when your witness Stephen was killed. I stood by and kept the coats they took off when they stoned him."

So he was at least involved in persecution, imprisoning, and physical beatings of Christians.

Yet something amazing happened to Saul. The Bible records it Acts 9:1–19. Read this section, and then answer the questions below.

What was the purpose of Saul's trip to Damascus?

_____

_____

_____

_____

_____

What happened that made Saul fall to the ground?

_____

_____

_____

_____

_____

After Saul heard his name called, and asked who was speaking to him, what answer did he receive?

_____

_____

_____

_____

_____

What did the men with Saul do? Would you have done any differently than they?

_____

_____

_____

What did the Lord instruct Paul to do?

_____

_____

_____

_____

_____

_____

_____

_____

_____

And what did Paul do?

_____

God took the sin of man, and used it for His glory.

_____

Now, you have been introduced but to a few of the important men in the Bible (and there are many more). But how does this tie into you being a godly man? Great question!

You have had the opportunity to see these men as to who they were; they were men of God who also, being human, failed as well. You have seen great travesties they have committed, yet they were still called by God to fulfill His work on this earth.

Abraham, a man called by God and who trusted God. God had never steered him wrong, yet Abraham decided not to trust God in His promise of delivering an heir. And what happened? He and Sarah set off a chain of events that hinder world peace even unto this very day. Two parties claim the right of inheritance to the land of Palestine and to the city of Jerusalem. Yet in the end, God forgave Abraham's transgressions (sins) and surely blessed him. He was a godly man who followed God's call on his life.

God took the sin of man and used it for His glory.

David, a man called by God and who sought to serve God and was blessed in many, many ways. He saw something he wanted that was not his, and that God did not give to him. Yet knowing he was wrong, he took it anyway. Then when it was obvious that his sin would show, he tried to fix it… not by confessing his sin, but by trying to hide it. It was such a failure that he had to have a man killed to hide that sin. Yet, in the end, God forgave his transgressions and surely blessed him. He was a godly man who followed God's call on his life.

God took the sin of man, and used it for His glory.

Paul, a man who trusted in the law, but not the God who gave the law. His allegiance was to a set of rules as a Jewish leader. He attacked and persecuted Christians; he beat them and even stood by as one of God's newly called preachers (Stephen), was stoned to death by an angry mob of non-Christians. Yet, in the end, God forgave his transgressions and surely blessed him. He was a godly man who followed God's call on his life.

God took the sin of man and used it for His glory.

So what is it, besides screwing up, that each of these men had in common? And how does that apply to you to make you, too, a godly man?

Each man, although he did terrible things, upon his repentance, obeyed. He became obedient. He did what God told him to do. Abraham continued on and founded nations due to his obedience. David continued on and through his family line, the Temple was built due to his obedience. Paul continued on and established the early church and missions and wrote letters that are used to this day, due to his obedience. And that makes them godly men. God took the sin of man, and used it for His glory.

And that also translates to *you*, even today. For no matter what transgressions you have made, you can now become obedient to God. And the first part of that, after salvation, is to put away that pornography. For a godly man doesn't view pornography. He honors and respects women and children. He gives it to God, as did Abraham, David, and Paul.

And once you begin to practice obedience, your godliness begins to grow. Because to be obedient to God means to not be obedient to the world. And though the road is not easy, you will find that being obedient to God is much more intriguing, for your life begins to change for the better. Your status in life may not change, but your acceptance, endurance, and desire to serve God will. And His light shining through you will be used by Him to bring others to Him.

God takes the sin of man and uses it for His glory. God takes the sin of *you* and uses it for His glory; if you will only repent and let Him.

Could God show Himself and make all be believers? Well, yes. And no. In the book of Revelation (the End Times), scripture says that *"For the Scriptures say, 'As surely as I live,' says the LORD, every knee will bend to me, and every tongue will confess and give praise to God.'"* (Romans 14:11). Revelation 19 tells us that Christ will appear on a white horse with an army of angels following. The description of Christ is extremely vivid. So there is your yes. If God as Father or Son shows Himself in His magnificent glory, then all will recognize and believe. Unfortunately, when this happens, individual eternities will have already been decided. It will be too late. But then, I also said, "and no." Because God has already shown Himself in the person of Christ, who not only was denied as Savior, but was crucified!

So you see, you, by accepting Christ, by accepting this challenge of refusing to use pornography and by choosing to become a vessel of Christ, well, you become a part of His army here on earth, until that time that He returns to restore glory and order. Although, God could indeed appear in all His glory and make all believe, He chooses to do it through His followers. And that, now, is you. You become a part of the body of Christ, which is called the church. And no, that does not mean a church building or a particular denomination. The church is not a building. The church is you. And me. And all followers of Christ.

I love you, brother; godly man. And I will stand by you in this fight.

God bless you, as you continue the journey through this study.

Record your memory verse for this lesson here:

Here is one last scripture. It is not a memory verse. It is words from Peter, Jesus' closest disciple. I believe it describes you, whether you are a new follower of Christ, or one who has been following Christ for some time:

³You have had enough in the past of the evil things that godless people enjoy—their immorality and lust, their feasting and drunkenness and wild parties, and their terrible worship of idols. ⁴Of course, your former friends are very surprised when you no longer join them in the wicked things they do, and they say evil things about you. ⁵But just remember that they will have to face God, who will judge everyone, both the living and the dead (1 Peter 4:3–5).

Your life has changed. If you have accepted Christ as your Lord and Savior, you are a new man. Those whom you used to party with, now may pull away from you. At first, that may bother you, but as you move away from them and into the caring and loving embrace of your brothers and sisters in Christ, you will find a much more comfortable, satisfying, and yes, a happier way.

God bless you, brother.

Here's a final thought for you, as you seek to become obedient to God, as all of these men were. It comes from Paul's letter to the Romans.

15So since God's grace has set us free from the law, does this mean we can go on sinning? Of course not! 16Don't you realize that whatever you choose to obey becomes your master? You can choose sin, which leads to death, or you can choose to obey God and receive His approval. 17Thank God! Once you were slaves of sin, but now you have obeyed with all your heart the new teaching God has given you. 18Now you are free from sin, your old master, and you become slaves to your new master, righteousness.

19I speak this way, using the illustration of slaves and masters, because it is easy to understand. Before, you let yourselves be slaves of impurity and lawlessness. Now you must choose to be slaves of righteousness so that you will become holy.

0In those days, when you were slaves of sin, you weren't concerned with doing what was right. 21And what was the result? It was not good, since now you are ashamed of the things you used to do, things that end in eternal doom. 22But now you are free from the power of sin and have become slaves of God. Now you do those things that lead to holiness and result in eternal life. 23For the wages of sin is death, but the free gift of God is eternal life through Christ Jesus our Lord.

(Romans 6:15–23)

Ending Prayer
Heavenly Father,

I am realizing more and more that I am a godly man. Teach me obedience, O Lord, that I may be the man that You desire me to be. I want to serve You, Lord, and to live my life so that others see You through me. Protect me from attacks by the Evil One, who will seek to destroy me and my ministry for You, O God. Make me strong in You, God, so that I may be of service to You.

In the Holy Name of Jesus Christ,
Amen

Awesome. You have come a long way already! Make sure to be in touch with your prayer partner this week. If he's not in the program, share with him about how you're striving to become a more godly man and ask him to keep you in prayer.

If you don't have a church home yet, how's your search going?

Is there anything else you learned during this lesson that you'd like to write down?

_____

_____

_____

_____

_____

_____

_____

She Is a Woman

³*The lips of an immoral woman are as sweet as honey,
and her mouth is smoother than oil.* ⁴*But the result is as
bitter as poison, sharp as a double-edged sword.* ⁵*Her feet
go down to death; her steps lead straight to the grave.*
⁷*So now, my sons; listen to me. Never stray from
what I am about to say: "Run from her!"*
—Proverbs 5:3–5; 7

In lesson 2, the study started out by talking about there being no middle ground. There is good, and there is evil. The same holds true in this lesson. Just as there are evil men out to destroy you and your relationship with God, there are also evil women out to do the same. All evil is driven by one being—Satan, also called the Evil One. And in all honesty, it is much easier for a man to walk away from the evil (worldly) influences of another man than it is for him to walk away from the evil (worldly) influences of a woman. And again, in all honesty, it is even harder to do so if she is beautiful and seductive.

Just like men, women face many of the same sin issues. While there is no doubt the way men and women think is so different, we are also alike. If we are made in the image of God, more so than the other creatures that inhabit the earth, can we be that different? So, women also face the issues of good vs. evil. And just like with men, sometimes it just seems easier to not resist the pull of the world while attempting to follow Christ. Sometimes it's just easier to "go with the flow." So women, too, face this dilemma:

Woman facing temptation, being pulled by good and evil.

Just as we said in lesson 2, let's say the same thing here, but change the word "man" to the word "woman."

The world teaches womanhood differently than the Bible teaches womanhood. While there are some similarities, the world takes God's law and perverts it to fit the goals of Satan, which is separation from God. Humanism is a great deception as well, teaching that humanity can conquer and solve all of mankind's problems, suggesting there is no need for God. Now, knowing that, who do you think is responsible for humanism? God? Or Satan?

Proverbs says in 4:23:

Above all else, guard your heart, for it affects everything you do.

Hey, let's make that this lesson's memory verse!

Why don't ya write that verse right here?!

_____

_____

_____

_____

Be careful who you choose. If you are already married, and she is not a Christian, do your best to bring her to Christ.

But now, let's add something else to this. If woman is, by direction of God, to be one in soul with her husband in Christ, then in addition to humanism, who do you think is responsible for feminism? God? Or Satan? Feminism, like humanism, goes *against* God's design and *with* the world's wishes. And who have we determined is the deceiver of this world? Yes, Satan.

Since we have cleared up that woman faces the same sin issues as man, let's look at those again. Just as Satan knows what entices you, he also knows what entices women, and yes, he will use every weapon in his arsenal against them as well.

Just like with man, woman faces the possibility of drug and alcohol addiction, pornography addiction, human trafficking, sex addiction, rampant sex with different (and sometimes multiple) partners. Sex with children. Sex with persons of the same sex, adultery, premarital sex, rape, robbery, theft, murder, idolatry, lust, deception, anger, hatred, brutality, conquest, greed, selfishness, meanness, arrogance, boastfulness.

Can you think of any other issues that you think may affect women in the worldly manner? Be nice.

_____

_____

_____

_____

Why does she tend to face the same sin issues and temptations as you? Because she is human.

Dictionary.com defines womanhood as the following: the state or quality of being a woman or being womanly; women collectively. Wow! That's even less of a description than what was given for the definition of manhood!

And maybe that describes why *worldly* women are just as lost (and maybe even more so) than worldly men! Let's see, now... worldly men who don't know Jesus, thus not knowing what their role is, mingling with worldly women who don't know their role either and have no one to lead by example. As Sheldon Cooper says in the hit show *Big Bang Theory,* bazinga! It's easy to see why everyone, male and female, is so lost, so confused, so deceived! Aha! Deceived! And who is the Great Deceiver?! Yes! Satan! Wow. That makes the answer so simple! Alas, though. Changing that world view is so difficult. Ugh!

So although we'll get to this in lesson VI, let's say it right here. *The reason that so many women (and men) are lost is because of you. And I. And all other men out there.* You will see that in lesson 4 that it is the responsibility of you and me, emblazoned in us at creation, to be the spiritual leaders here on earth. And I hope, that upon looking at the current state of the world, you would agree with me that we have been terrible at our job. Because the world is a disaster. Oh, yeah, there are good parts all around. In general, though, it appears to be falling apart. And that rests on the shoulders of you, me, and all the other men.

The world wants women to be beautiful and sexy, thin and hot, seductive. Lara Croft. BloodRayne. Princess Leia. Daenerys Targaryen.

All of them are strong, beautiful, and sexy, as the world would portray them. Now, there's nothing wrong with women being strong and beautiful. The world portrays often that they have no need of men; for they can do all things that men can do. It empowers women, while belittling men. Well now, who do you think would want for that to happen?! Yep, that ol' Satan again.

You see, women should be empowered, as men should. Not through power, beauty, strength, and sexiness. But through God. God is the one who empowers eternally. And God bestows those things in His way.

List a few things that you see as how the world wants you to envision a woman: _____

_____

_____

_____

_____

_____

So you see, women, like men, are fallen creatures. But they are no different than you are, for Adam and Eve fell together. While some seem to blame woman for The Fall, you will learn that, in the end, it was an equal Fall. And in reality, Adam is more to blame than is Eve.

It is the responsibility of you and I to show proper leadership, as God designed, to empower woman to become one with Jesus Christ. Remember, she is lost as well. It is our job to deliver where Adam failed—leadership. Oh, it's going to be so awesome when you "get it"!

Let's get ready to move to the next section; but first… yep. Write your memory verse for this week here:

_____
_____
_____
_____
_____
_____
_____

And as always, end this session with a prayer.

Heavenly Father,

I admit it, God. I just don't know a lot about women. Especially women of the world. I know what the world wants me to see. It wants me to want them in an unclean way. It wants me to lust, and entices me to treat women disrespectfully. Lord, I pray not only that you open my eyes to what a woman of God looks like, but also for those women who have been deceived by Satan and pulled away from You, O God. Be with them, let them be led to salvation in Jesus.

For it in His name I ask these things.

Amen.

Okay. Honesty here. Continue praying for guidance. Love your woman (wife). I'm going no further on this one. I don't want to get in trouble with my own boss lady.

Lesson V

She Is a Godly Woman

²⁰She extends a helping hand to the poor
and opens her arms to the needy.
²⁵She is clothed with strength and dignity, and she laughs with no fear
of the future. ²⁶When she speaks, her words are wise, and kindness is the
rule when she gives instructions. ²⁷She carefully watches all that goes on
in her household and does not have to bear the consequences of laziness.
²⁸Her children stand and bless her. Her husband
praises her: ²⁹"There are many virtuous and capable
women in the world, but you surpass them all!"
³⁰Charm is deceptive, and beauty does not last; but a woman
who fears the Lord will be greatly praised. ³¹Reward her for
all she has done. Let her deeds publicly declare her praise.
—Proverbs 31:20, 25–31

The passage quoted here is intended to describe a wife of noble character. But I do sincerely believe that we can ascribe this to any woman
who seeks to be a woman of God, a servant of God. The world, as was
said in the previous lesson, wants you to look only, as verse 30 starts
out, seeing only the charm and beauty (dare I say, "seductiveness").

OUT OF THE DARKNESS

But God's Word is vividly clear in the last statement of verse 30, "but a woman who fears the Lord will be greatly praised." Remember, beauty does not last; it is fleeting. At least, physical beauty. Inner beauty lasts a lifetime.

My mother was a godly woman. She feared the Lord, and she was blessed by her children. I remember when she died in 2013, one of my brothers told me that he was concerned about me and thought maybe I didn't care that Mom had passed. I asked him why he felt that way; he replied that it was because I had not shed a tear. I smiled and told him that my time would come for tears, but really, I asked him, "How can I be sad when mama is in the presence of God?" Her beauty reigned all of her life.

Yes, physical beauty does not last, but inner beauty of a woman who fears the Lord is eternal.

And I want to go ahead and introduce your memory verse for this week. Yes, it is indeed the one we have just discussed.

Charm is deceptive, and beauty does not last; but a woman who fears the Lord is greatly praised (Proverbs 31:30).

Write it here:

_____

_____

_____

_____

A godly woman is a strong woman. A strong woman indeed.

_____

_____

Let's look at some of these strong women and the service they offered to the Lord their God. Let's look at how a woman of God should appear, despite what the world says.

If you're going to pull a woman from the Bible to talk about, the first one to speak of would have to be Ruth. She was so important and so humble that God ensured she got a book in the Bible! Now, that's pretty snazzy, if ya ask me!

Ruth's story is found in the Old Testament, just after the book of Judges. In fact, it is believed that her time on earth was during the time of the Judges. What her story shows is how loyalty and humility are traits that God desires, and He rewarded her justly. You see, Ruth was not an Israelite, meaning that she was looked down upon by those of the Jewish faith.

Read Ruth 1:1–5 then share what happened in those verses

_____

_____

_____

_____

_____

_____

_____

_____

_____

_____

_____

_____

Ruth returned to Israel with Naomi, despite Naomi's pleas for her to stay in her own homeland. Naomi didn't want to keep Ruth from remarrying, but Ruth insisted on staying with Naomi. Ruth, upon arriving in Bethlehem, finds work in the fields of Boaz, who is a relative of Naomi. Boaz treats her well as a result of the love and loyalty that Ruth showed to her mother-in-law. Boaz falls for Ruth and they marry. This is important. And you can learn why by reading the last part of Ruth. (4:13–22). Now, record verses 21–22 here: (I've helped you out a little)

21 _____

_____
22
_____

_____

_____

Ah, do you see it? Ruth was the great grandmother of David! And yes, that's King David whom we spoke of in lesson 3! Whoa! See how God works? Kind of amazing isn't it? Whoop Whoop!

_____

_____

Another important woman of God is Esther. She, too, is in the Old Testament. Her book is just before the book of Job. Wait… is that Job, as in Job's Warriors?! Why, yes it is! But that comes along later!

Back to Esther. Her story takes place during the Exile, when the Israelites had been disobedient to God and He allowed their capture by the Babylonians. They were taken to Persia. Xerxes became King of Persia (formerly Babylonia). Xerxes was married to a beautiful woman, his queen, Vashti. He wanted all to gaze upon her beauty and summoned her. She refused. This angered Xerxes, and upon the counsel of his advisors, he banished her and sought out a new queen. Xerxes, having no clue that Esther was a Jew, chose her to be the queen. (Okay, it really wasn't quite that simple, but I'm just trying to shorten the story!) Mordecai, Esther's uncle, was a servant of the king; when he learned of an assassination plot against Xerxes, he passed the information to Esther. When she relayed the info to Xerxes, she gave Mordecai credit. When it was found to be true, the plotters were hanged. To make a somewhat long story short, and to show her role as a woman of God, Esther played an integral role. You see, Haman, the prime minister serving under Xerxes, hated the Jews. He devised a plan to have the king make a decree to kill them. Esther, whom Xerxes loved and trusted, had to divulge her nationality to the king. Based on his decree, that meant death for her; if she remained silent, she would not die.

Read Esther chapters 5 through 7. I'm not going to ask you to share what you read here. I really think that after the background was laid above, you will certainly get the picture. Esther was a woman of God, who risked her own life to obey God's calling to save His people.

_____

_____

The next woman of God I want to mention was not originally a woman of God at all. But God used her to do what He needed done. Her name was Rahab. You can find her story in Joshua 2. Rahab was a prostitute. And you thought prostitutes were only good for satisfying the lustful and sexual desires of men. I'm sure that Rahab was thought of in much the same light as modern prostitutes are— not very pleasant thoughts. But God can and does use anyone He chooses. (I hope you are beginning to see that with some of the people we've already discussed, and from the stirring that God is causing in your own heart. For I am sure that you, like me, have thought yourself unworthy of God's love. I hope you are starting to feel how wrong you are. He does love you, so much that He gave His Son for you.)

I hate to ask you to read yet again, but read you must. Joshua 2. See how God took a woman who was not respected by her community and made her invaluable.

Give a brief summary here, but also add how that inspires you that obedience to God is so important. Include what God is saying to *you*.

_____

_____

_____

_____

_____

_____

_____

_____

_____

_____

_____

_____

_____

_____

_____

_____

_____

_____

But there is another interesting tidbit of information about Rahab of which you are probably not aware. First, you learned that she was a prostitute, a "line of work" not looked well upon at all in these ancient times. How she got into prostitution can only be speculated, but there is something that you really need to be aware of here as to how God works.

I really need you to turn to the gospel of Matthew in your Bible. And I want you to read Matthew 1:4–6. It is part of the genealogy of Jesus.

Do you see it? Ruth, introduced above, was the great grand-mother of King David! And Rahab was the mother of Boaz, Ruth's husband! Wow! Rahab, a prostitute who hid the spies of Israel, became the great-great-grandmother of the King of Israel! Whoa! But wait! I pointed out that this is the genealogy of Jesus! Rahab was directly in the line of Jesus Christ, who came to save you from your sin!

God took the sin of man, and used it for His glory!

Do you realize how much God loves you?

So you've seen some godly women from the Old Testament. We have to discuss at least *one* from the New Testament! Wouldn't you agree? I thought you would. But alas, I can think of two that *need* to be mentioned.

The first one is Mary, the very mother of Jesus Christ. The mother of the Messiah. This was a woman whose faith was and is beyond question. She was young, some say as young as fourteen, others say around sixteen (things were a lot different back then). However, her age is really not relevant. It is her faith that is out front here. She was engaged to Joseph. To be pregnant, when she was believed to be a virgin, had to really set some people back! Even Joseph was hesitant to marry her. But let's look at what happened.

Of the four gospels that begin the New Testament, only the gospel of Luke includes the story of Mary. It begins in Luke 1 verse 26. The Angel of the Lord, Gabriel, appears to Mary and informs her that she has been chosen to deliver the Lord Jesus. Mary is confused, but she listens, and is obedient. The only question she asks Gabriel is how she, a virgin, can be pregnant. But she accepts his answer and declares this,

²⁶*"I am the Lord's servant, and I am willing to accept whatever He wants. May everything you have said come true." And then the angel left* (Luke1:38).

You can probably imagine the difficult time she had, being young, unmarried, and pregnant. But Joseph stood by her. And she was indeed blessed with the birth of the One who would provide salvation for humanity. *"I am the Lord's servant."* Mary, mother of Jesus, was indeed a woman of God.

The last woman of God we'll discuss is Mary Magdalene. She is mentioned in every gospel; Luke and Mark say that Jesus cast seven demons from her. She became a devout follower of Christ, as witnessed in Luke 8:1–2,

¹*Not long afterward Jesus began a tour of the nearby cities and villages to announce the Good News concerning the Kingdom of God. He took His twelve disciples with Him,* ²*along with some women he had healed and from whom He had cast out evil spirits. Among them were Mary Magdalene, from whom He had cast out seven demons;*

Mary Magdalene followed Jesus throughout His ministry. She was obedient to His call to her. She was there at His crucifixion, and she was one of the women present when the tomb was found empty. Read Luke 24:10. Now, go back and read Luke 8:3.

Who do you see that was with Mary Magdalene on both occasions?

_____ While we only spoke of Mary Magdalene here, you see that Joanna was also a devout follower.

So you see, women of God have been present, like men of God, since the inception of the Creation. And in the next session, you're going to learn all about *your calling* as a man of God.

And you are ready!

Write your memory verse here again:

_____

_____

_____

_____

Let's end this session with a prayer!

Gracious Father,

Teach me to look for Your qualities in both men and women. But Lord, as I enter the next lesson, prepare me for and teach me how to be a man that empowers women in You.

In Your Name I pray,

Amen.

How's your journaling, reading, and prayer going? How are you holding up in the study itself? Good, I hope. Don't forget to keep in touch with your prayer partner. You have been introduced to what a godly woman may look like. Can a woman find Christ and live a godly life without a man? Absolutely. But it's your role to provide an example of Godliness. So pray for guidance in that area.

Have you found a church yet?

Do you have any questions after this section? Write them down. Send 'em to us at our website if you need to.

Lesson VI

Your Calling as a Man of God

As I was writing this Bible study, I asked my wife, Melinda, a question. I asked her how she felt all of those years as I led her into acting out the sexual fantasies that I had shared with her. I remember her asking me one time, many years ago, what my fantasies were. I hesitated, asking her if she was sure she wanted to know. I then shared them with her. I don't know that she intended me to take those fantasies to the level that I did, as I said in the introduction to this study. But I never really asked either, because I felt that I was given permission.

So when I recently asked her how she felt about all those fantasies, she didn't seem too moved by the question. Expecting her to say that she felt dirty, or shamed, I asked pointedly if that was, indeed, how she had felt. Her answer completely surprised me. And while some men would think her answer was a great answer, I was even more taken aback than I expected to be. For she did not give me the standard answer that I expected. Instead her answer was that they never bothered her because she "felt safe" with me. I said a moment ago that some men would love that answer! It gives them the chance to act out fantasies with a woman willing to participate. And the man I was over five years ago would have loved this answer as well. But now, as a man who follows Christ and does his best to be a man of God, I find that answer disturbing. She "felt safe" with me? What kind of man did that make me? A man of the world (evil)? Or a man of God? Yes, the correct answer is a man of the world! My wife "felt safe." What kind of safety was I giving her? I was leading her down the path of destruction! That's part of what disturbed me about her answer.

But here's the real kicker:

> [7] *In the same way, you husbands must give **honor** to your wives.*
> *treat your wife with understanding as you live together.*
> *she may be weaker than you are, but she is your equal partner in God's*
> *gift of new life. Treat her as you should so your prayers*
> *will not be hindered.* (1 Peter 3:7)

Honor? Was I honoring Melinda by making her a *token*, an *image*, an *object* of my desires?! What a joke I was for a man! That is not a man! A man takes his wife by the hand, recognizing that she is the image of God, and treats her with *respect* and *honor*! Remember the scripture early on (a memory verse) from Psalm 86:11 where we ask God to "*Grant me purity of heart, that I may honor You.* Do you really think we *honor* God by *dishonoring* our wife?!

The Greek word used for the word *understanding* is gnosin (γνωσίν), which means "knowledge." Gnosin comes from gnosis (γνωσίς), translated as "a knowing," "knowledge" or "acquaintance with" a person. In other words, treat your wife as one you are acquainted with; not a stranger or a threat.

Record times you have *dishonored* your wife (or fiancé, or girlfriend):

_____

_____

_____

_____

_____

_____

_____

_____

_____

_____

_____

_____

Now, record how you can reverse that and begin to **honor** your wife (or fiancé, or girlfriend):

_____

_____

_____

_____

_____

_____

_____

_____

_____

_____

_____

Writing things down, where you can see them, can certainly be revealing, can't it?

_____

This lesson will be talking about your *calling* as a man of God. You've seen how you are to *be* a man of God. But now, what are you supposed to do with it? If there is a place where the church (the body of Christ) has failed *miserably,* it is the aspect of who you are as a man of God *and* your calling as a man of God. Don't believe it? Walk into a church any day and just say that you'd like to ask how many men in the church use pornography! Better yet, ask it at some church function! Whoa! You will probably get run out of the place! I am constantly amazed at how hard the church fights homosexuality, but doesn't want to address pornography! Of course, I do understand the reluctance. For most people, to hear someone say they are addicted to pornography (or that they even look at it at all) is like saying they are homosexual! Because any man who has looked at porn knows it leads to masturbation. And we certainly can't talk about that! In all honesty, the great majority of wives and other women see masturbation and perusing pornography as some type of perversion. *It's time we stopped looking at it as a perversion. It is an evil, a sin, that Satan uses to separate man from God and man from woman. Period.* Now, don't beat yourself up over it, and don't feel ashamed. *You* are not a bad person; you are simply manipulated by the world. As you begin to try and become more godly, Satan will tempt you to the utmost. Quite honestly, you will fall short and give in to your desires. But as you grow in Christ and learn more about repentance, it will become easier to reject these desires for the holiness of God. Trust me. Been there, done that. And guess what? Satan, when I'm in my most quiet or alone times, tells me, "Go ahead. Don't worry about it." And I have learned to get up and get busy and pray as I do so.

Most churches are also reluctant to speak about human trafficking, although many will at least acknowledge it and maybe even have some type of outreach. But there are two problems here as well. First, if it is acknowledged, then something must be done, so it's easier to ignore. Second, most can understand and be greatly appalled at a child who is trafficked, but an adult? Most see adult prostitution as a choice. Of course, we'll get more into both of these in the next couple of lessons.

But let's look at your calling as a man of God. That's the beginning of getting past this stuff and beginning not only to help others get through it (with Christ), but also to begin to defend the honor of women everywhere!

Put on your armor, man of God! You're going to need it! Ephesians 6:10–18. Read it and write it down here!

_____

_____
_____
_____
_____
_____
_____
_____
_____
_____
_____
_____
_____
_____
_____
_____
_____
_____

Good deal. Now, move forward, man of God. And enter the battle.

_____

Let's start by looking at various scripture references. We talked in lesson 3 about you as a man of God. As you recall, we started when

Noah exited the ark and that man (humanity) was again given charge of the world. But from there, we know that the world turned evil again, as it had after Adam and Eve sinned in the Garden (The Fall). We saw how Abraham, David, and Paul, although men of God, fell short of God's glory through their own various sins. And we related that to you. If you'll recall this statement from page 31, *"And that also translates to you, even today. For no matter what transgressions you have made, you can now become obedient to God. And the first part of that, after salvation, is to put away that pornography. For a godly man doesn't view pornography. He honors and respects women and children. He gives it to God, as did Abraham, David, and Paul."*

All right! Here we go! Ya ready? Hold on to the reins, brother!

²⁶ That is why God abandoned them to their shameful desires. Even the women turned against the natural way to have sex and instead indulged in sex with each other.

²⁷ And the men, instead of having normal sexual relationships, with women, burned with lust for each other. Men did shameful things with other men and, as a result, suffered within themselves the penalty they so richly deserved (Romans 1:26–27).

Uh-oh. That kind of blows things up, doesn't it? Those desires you may have had for seeing two women together, well, shucks. God kind of puts a damper on that doesn't He?

Okay, so how does this affect your calling as a man of God? Good question! And there are lots of ways, some of which we will definitely discuss! But hear this, the next few lines of that passage of Romans:

²⁸ When they refused to acknowledge God, He <u>abandoned</u> them to their evil minds and let them do things that should never be done. ²⁹ Their lives became full of every kind of wickedness, sin, greed, hate, envy, murder, fighting, deception, malicious behavior, and gossip. ³⁰ They are backstabbers, haters of God, insolent, proud, and boastful. They are forever inventing new ways of sinning and are disobedient to their par-

ents. [31] *They refuse to understand, break their promises, and are heartless and unforgiving.* [32] *They are fully aware of God's death penalty for those who do these things, yet they go right ahead and do them anyway. And, worse yet, they encourage others to do them, too* (Romans 1:28–32).

Paul is saying that by practicing sexual immorality, it will lead to all of these other sinful lifestyles. And it includes pornography. You see, porn is very dark. And darkness is where Satan lives and thrives. No matter where you are or were in your pornography viewing, darkness rules. No matter where you are in your use of pornography, one or more of the sin attributes listed in this latest passage are part of who you are. You know it; just as I faced some of those very same demons, and other men before you have faced some of them. I'll list mine for you right here. I suffered from *hate.* I suffered from *envy.* I suffered from *deception.* I suffered from *malicious behavior (I was mean).* I suffered from *gossip.* I was a *backstabber.* I was a *hater of God.* I was *proud* and I was *boastful.* I had trouble keeping *promises.* I was *cold-hearted* and I was *unforgiving.* I was also aware of God's penalty for these sins, but I did not care. Perhaps you are in the same boat. Or perhaps you just didn't know. You do now.

Record here which of the above sin attributes describe you.

_____

_____

_____

_____

_____

_____

_____

_____

_____

_____

What is the purpose of the above scriptures from Romans? Part of your calling as a man of God is to *not* be the above type of man!

For you know that your job is to protect, honor, respect. And none of those attributes listed above even offer a glimpse of godly attributes.

Let's look a little further at your directions from God as to how you're supposed to act as one of His men. Read Leviticus 18:6–17 and 20–23. You don't have to write anything here. Instead, use a highlighter (or pen to underline) each person you are not to have sex with. And yes, obedience to this is being a man of God. But don't fret, if you have asked God for forgiveness and have repented of any of these you *have* had sex with, then your obedience is beginning. So don't beat yourself up. You are (or can be) forgiven. Begin living your calling as a man of God now.

⁹Don't you know that those who do wrong will have no share in the Kingdom of God? Don't fool yourselves. Those who indulge in sexual sin, who are idol worshipers, adulterers, male prostitutes, homosexuals, ¹⁰thieves, greedy people, drunkards, abusers, and swindlers—none of these will have a share in the Kingdom of God (1 Corinthians 6:9–10).

Interesting. Again, this leads off with the corruption of sexual sin. I wonder why sex is such a big deal and seems to be an integral part of leading to other sinful behaviors. Hmmmm…

Do you remember lesson 1? If not, turn back and take a look. "*In the beginning*"—whoa. I'm taking you back to that? Yep. Afraid so.

²³"At last!" Adam exclaimed. "She is part of my own flesh and bone! She will be called 'woman,' because she was taken out of a man." ²⁴This explains why a man leaves his father and mother and is joined to his wife, and the two are united into one (Genesis 2:23–24).

and

³Some Pharisees came and tried to trap Him with this question: "Should a man be allowed to divorce his wife for any reason?" ⁴"Haven't you read the Scriptures?" Jesus replied. "They record that from the beginning 'God made them male and female.' ⁵And He said, 'This explains why a man leaves his father and mother and is joined to his wife, and the two are united into one.' [6]*Since they are no longer two but one, let no one separate them, for God has joined them together"* (Matthew 19:3–6)

It should be obvious to you that sex was defined by God to be enjoyed within the confines of marriage and not outside of marriage. Thus, you can see pretty quickly that when sex is practiced outside of the way God designed it to be, it is a catalyst for other sinful behavior. For who do you think is in the midst of non-marital sex? God? Or Satan? Interesting, isn't it? Have you ever asked yourself, "man, where did I screw up so bad to be in the life of porn (or insert other sinful lifestyle(s) here)?" Well, now you know. It started with satisfying *your* desires, and not the desires that God has for you. All of us who have spit in God's face have done the same things.

Wow. Just as you've already learned (hopefully), you cannot place your faith, your needs, your desires, your necessity to be a man in pornography or other dishonorable treatment of woman. You just can't. The "deep within the center" that Eldridge is talking about is the Holy Spirit. Let your strength come from deep inside (the Holy Spirit), rather than outside sources—pornography, non-marital sex, alcohol, drugs, or any host of things! Jesus Christ is your strength and He will lead your calling as a man of God!

In the book *Wild at Heart,* John Eldridge says it this way, "*Most men want the maiden without any sort of cost to themselves. They want all the joys of the beauty without any of the woes of the battle. This is the sinister nature of pornography—enjoying the woman at her expense. Pornography is what happens when a man insists on being energized by a woman, he uses her to get a feeling that he is a man. It is a false strength, as I've said, because it depends on an outside source rather than emanating from deep within his center.*
Eldridge, John, *Wild at Heart,* Thomas Nelson Publishers, Nashville, TN, 2001, 2010, 189

A few years ago, I was in the hospital for an extended stay and had some major surgery. I was a believer in Christ, working on becoming a follower of Christ (I highly recommend reading *Not a Fan* by Kyle Idleman and *Radical* by David Platt, info included in the back of the study). But my faith wavered. I had never been so sick and was questioning why God was allowing this after I had submitted to Him following running in sin for 30 years. I became reliant on my wife, Melinda, rather than on God. And while Melinda is everything to me, she does not have the ability to save my soul. Only one person has that ability—the man Jesus Christ. It doesn't matter in what you place your faith—a woman, a friend, a porn star, alcohol, etc. None can save you. Only Jesus can provide salvation. All else is idolatry. Anything, and I mean anything, that you put above God is, in fact, idolatry. There is nothing at all wrong with having a love for things. That is our nature.

What occurred in the hospital overall is a story for another time, but it was amazing and it was to be part of my journey to increase my faith in Jesus.

Idolatry is defined *Merriam-Webster Dictionary* as "the worship of a picture or object as a god."

It is when we place "things," or even, "ideas," *above* God, or we make it an object(s) of *worship* that it becomes a problem. When you will do anything for that particular car, for that particular person, or for that next sexual satisfaction, that it becomes idolatry. And God forbids idolatry early on. Remember the Ten Commandments? Hmmmm... no. 1... you shall have no other gods (idols) before Me. That's pretty clear, isn't it? Yeah, I think so too.

My point? Pornography was no longer my idol. What I didn't realize until my hospital stay was that I didn't replace pornography with God, as I thought I had. No, I had made my wife to be my god. But God will not accept even that. You are to love your wife, but *He is to be your God*. Period.

With all this said, this is also a great time to bring in your memory verse for this lesson. It should be an easy enough verse! Since your main reason for doing this Bible study is your addiction to, or desire for pornography, and you have now identified porn as an idol, here it is! You'll love this one!

So my dear friends, flee from the worship of idols (1 Corinthians 10:14).

Now, write down here:

_____

_____

_____

See? Wasn't that an easy one? But it is oh so important to your walk with God.

This section, like lesson 3, is a little long. So if you choose, this is a great place to stop, and pick up next week. Get some rest. While being a man of God and finding your calling as a man of God is the best reward available, Satan sure does challenge you the whole way.

---

³Take control of what I say, O Lord,
and keep my lips sealed.
⁴Don't let me lust for evil things;
Don't let me participate in the acts of wickedness.
don't let me share in the delicacies
of those who do evil (Psalm 141: 3–4)

Another one of many scriptures in the Word of God that teach about your calling as a man of God. Read that one again, and then just let it sit a minute. Do you realize what it's saying to you? You see, as you step out on faith and into the presence of almighty God, you will long to be this type of man. You will long to do all you can, peacefully, ethically, and legally (within the confines of man's law) to do things of God, rather than of the world (evil). And you will long to reach others so that they too, may find the same joy that you have found. That's what men of God do—avoid wickedness while doing their best to share their faith.

And that is what you are called to do, man of God. And you start by cleaning yourself up spiritually. Once that's done, God can work on the rest of you.

By the way, that Psalm you just read above? It's credited to a guy by the name of David. Yes, as in King David. Amazing how God works, isn't it? Remember that David fell—big time. Yet here he is, asking for purity. Just as you are doing now.

All right. You're ready to get into this "calling" thing. I've done a lot of talking about the "calling," but you want the meat of what it means to find your "calling as a man of God." Quite honestly, what you're about to do is only the basics, it's only the tip of the iceberg. For as you move forward in your faith, you will find your true calling as a man of God. But you must have some of the basics down. Your knowledge of your calling as a man of God will increase as you grow in Christ. At the end of this study, you will be given some information to help you.

Here we go! Are you ready? Let's learn what the basics of your calling are!

Todd Wagner, pastor of Watermark Community Church in Dallas, Texas offers these *5 Characteristics of a Godly Man.*[1]

---

[1] http://wordsfromwags.com/how-to-be-a-godly-man/

1. STEP UP: Lead. Initiate. Be a man of action. Assume it is your job and your moment. Hate apathy. Reject passivity.
2. SPEAK OUT: Silence in the midst of sin is a sin. Be courageous. Fear God, not man. Speak the truth in love.
3. STAND STRONG: Don't give in when you are challenged, attacked, or criticized.
4. STAY HUMBLE: Be vigilant against pride. Get the log out of your eye. Don't think less of yourself, think of yourself less.
5. SERVE THE KING: Seek first His Kingdom, His glory, His righteousness. Hope in the eternal. Live for a greater reward.

I think these characteristics are right on target. I encourage you to go to the footnoted website and check 'em out.

If I could sum up all the above characteristics in one word, it would be this: LEADERSHIP. God created you, sir, to be a leader in His world. Some will take objection to this, and I'm sorry they feel this way, but God created man first. It's that plain and simple. And it's Biblical. Woman was part of the plan all along, but she was created from man. And things get backwards when the woman leads. Now, yes, there are times when she does indeed lead certain areas; perhaps she's a single mom, perhaps she runs a business or even a ministry geared toward women (men can still learn from such ministries—those types of things.

You are to be the leader of your household. And that means if you're married, or planning to be married (dating or engaged), then you are to be the leader. But let's clear something up before we go any further! Some men misinterpret this leadership role. Even today, you can see this in churches. Men think they are to *dominate*! And nothing could be more wrong. God did not make woman from man's head for her to dominate, nor did He make her from the foot to be dominated (trampled upon). No, He made her from the side to be an equal partner. Man's leadership of woman comes in the spiritual realm. For if we lead properly, we help lead her to a meaningful relationship with Jesus Christ. Can she have a meaningful relationship with Christ without you? Absolutely, she can. But God designed it so that *you* can make her relationship with Him even more meaningful!

Remember this from the opening of this lesson?

> *[7] In the same way, you husbands must give **honor** to your wives.*
> *treat your wife with understanding as you live together.*
> *she may be weaker than you are, but she is your equal partner in God's*
> *gift of new life. Treat her as you should so your prayers*
> *will not be hindered.* (1 Peter 3:7)

Personally, I would like to know where in that passage does it say male leadership is domination? It doesn't say anything at all about domination. Nothing. Not a. Zilch.

But is says a lot about leadership.

Honor.
Understanding. LEADERSHIP
Equal Partner
Prayers

Are you getting that? The last word—prayers. God says that in order for your prayers to be heard unhindered, you had better treat your wife right. And in all honesty, you should treat all women right. Granted, your wife should always—let me repeat that—*always* be on a higher plane than other women; but you should still respect other women.

And I'm sorry to report that gazing at naked women in porn magazines or movies *does not honor them*, and it certainly *doesn't honor your wife*. Furthermore, it *doesn't honor God*. Plain and simple. Period. Nor does gazing at suggestively clothed women in *any* magazine. Period. And you're going to learn some things about pornography in the next lesson that I hope bursts any bubbles you still may have about porn.

Leadership. That is your primary calling as a man of God.

Leadership. Something in which man has failed since the beginning. Remember back early in this study when you learned about The Fall? Here is where it really comes to show how we as the male have failed in our role as leader of God's world. During the description of The Fall, there is a key statement made. At the end of Genesis 3:6, here is that statement, "*So she ate some of the fruit. She also gave some to her husband, who was with her*. Did you get that? History has blamed Eve for The Fall. But, Adam *was with her*. That is the first recorded event where man failed in his calling to be spiritual leader. Satan attacked God's ultimate creation, that which was created in the very image of God, in an attempt to separate humanity from God. And he succeeded in his attempt; because Adam fell short. Adam's job was to step up and not dominate Eve, but to lead her by example. Adam was to stand by her, to protect her from the deception that Satan was using; but instead Adam chose to do nothing. And then what happened later? Do you remember? God came looking for them, knowing what had happened. And what did Adam do? Genesis 3:12 records that when God asked Adam if he ate the fruit, Adam said, "*Yes, but it was the woman You gave me who brought me the fruit and I ate it."* What? Adam threw Eve right under the bus! You know the term we guys often use to challenge each other? We say, "Man up." Did Adam man up? Heck no. He wimped out when Satan approached Eve and then wimped out again, even *blaming* Eve, for the sin.

And we, gentlemen, still do the same thing today. Sad, isn't it?

There is another reason, though, that Leadership is such a big deal. In order to lead, you must learn to serve. Heed these words from our Lord and Savior,

> *"For even the Son of Man came not to be served*
> *but to serve others and to give his life*
> *as a ransom for many"* (Matthew 20:28).

Let me ask you a question. How many men do you personally know who are successful in life? And of those men, how many pretty much expect to be served? Maybe they're good bosses who treat their people fairly, but how do they act in a restaurant? At a store? Or here's a good one—how does he act in a bar? Any place where service people work? Now, read Jesus' words again above.

And this is why your Leadership as a man is so important—when you have a devout spiritual relationship with God, you allow others to do the same. You are leading by example. Your goal is to be Christlike. And you lead by serving.

Paul says, in his letter to the Philippians,

"³Don't be selfish; don't live to make a good impression on others. Be humble, thinking of others as better than yourself. ⁴Don't think only about your own affairs, but be interested in others, too, and what they are doing. ⁵Your attitude should be the same that Christ Jesus had. ⁶Though He was God, He did not demand and cling to His rights as God. ⁷He made Himself nothing; He took the humble position of a slave and appeared in human form. ⁸And in human form he obediently humbled Himself even further by dying a criminal's death on a cross. (Keep in mind that another word for slave, is servant)[2] (Philippians 2:3–8)

Express here what this is saying to you. Now, don't be too hard on yourself. That's not what all of this is about. This is about true freedom, found only in Jesus Christ!

_____

_____

_____

_____

_____

_____

_____

_____

Do you see any changes that you may need to make?

_____

_____

_____

_____

---

[2]   Parentheses mine.

If you are a married man, being Christlike is also extremely important in your marriage. Because, you see, *you* are the key to your wife's relationship with Christ. Oh, of course, she can have that without you, but because you are in a God ordained relationship as husband and wife, it is your calling to help her release herself. And this happens based on how you act!

Here's what Paul says in the letter to Ephesians,

"²³ For a husband is the head of his wife as Christ is the head of the church. He is the Savior of his body, the church. ²⁴ As the church submits to Christ, so you wives should submit to your husbands in everything.

²⁵ For husbands, this means love your wives, just as Christ loved the church. He gave up his life for her ²⁶ to make her holy and clean, washed by the cleansing of God's word. ²⁷ He did this to present her to himself as a glorious church without a spot or wrinkle or any other blemish. Instead, she will be holy and without fault. ²⁸ In the same way, husbands ought to love their wives as they love their own bodies. For a man who loves his wife actually shows love for himself. ²⁹ No one hates his own body but feeds and cares for it, just as Christ cares for the church. ³⁰ And we are members of his body.

³¹ As the Scriptures say, "A man leaves his father and mother and is joined to his wife, and the two are united into one. ³² This is a great mystery, but it is an illustration of the way Christ and the church are one. ³³ So again I say, each man must love his wife as he loves himself, and the wife must respect her husband. (Ephesians 5:23–33)

The scary thing in a Bible study is what the reader sees when he reads it. Some men will focus in on a few phrases, such as "wives should submit," or the wife "must respect her husband." But before you get hooked on those phrases, look at the whole passage again. In reality, the instructions are mainly to you, gentlemen. Not her. It is telling *you* how to act, in order for her to act accordingly. It's very simple. Love your wives as Christ loved the church. He gave up His life for the church to make her (the church) holy and clean. Whew. That's hardcore stuff, guys.

Go back and read Matthew 20:28. Christ came not to be served, but to serve. And to give His life as a ransom. So guess what. Your wife learns to serve by your example. You serve Christ. You serve her. You serve your children. You serve your neighborhood. You serve your community. You serve the world. You give up your life in "the world" in order to serve God. You do this, and she will indeed respect you, if she, too, is a Christian. It's that simple. It really is. Women who are Christian want a man who will lead in Christ. And that's how you lead—by following Christ and by making Christ the center of your marriage (verses 31 and 32 above). Here are a few tips to help you learn this leadership role:

Read your Bible daily. Make time for it. Let nothing interrupt it.

Pray daily.

Read your Bible with her.

Pray daily with her.

Pray with your children.

Find a church, if you don't already have one, and begin to attend as a family.

If you haven't been baptized, make that a priority. Baptism is a public statement of your faith.

If you're not yet married, these same principles apply. If you are engaged to be married, or are dating someone, always treat them with honor and respect. Follow the same habits of study and prayer. If you're totally single with no prospects in your immediate future, or if you are dating occasionally, these same principles still apply.

You see, it's about your relationship with Jesus Christ. And as all people, not just the ladies, see your relationship with Christ, they will see your sincerity and your maturity and leadership qualities in Him begin to grow.

So after all this, you can see that your calling as a man of God boils down, really, to two main characteristics—service, which leads to leadership. You are to serve Christ, which in turn causes you to serve others. This in turn gives you leadership. And that is who God calls you to be—a leader.

Get away from the world. It is selfish. And it makes you selfish. Using women (and others, for that matter) for your pleasure or for your gain is selfish. Selfishness is of Satan. Selfishness is sinful. You, through Christ, are cleansed of sin; therefore you are called to live differently. You are called to be like Christ—who Himself was a Leader who led through service, even unto crucifixion.

And now, you are part of the mightiest army that has, or ever will, be upon this earth. If you accept the challenge, you become a warrior. A warrior of God. And all men like to be warriors. More about warriors in lesson 9.

Record your memory verse here:

_____
_____
_____
_____

Ending Prayer
O, Holy Father,

As I learn more about You, I become stronger. Lord, I never understood my role in this world. And while I still have so much more to learn about You, and about my role in your calling to me, I can begin to feel Your Spirit working in me. Lord, teach me your ways, so that I may truly live according to your truth. O God, yes, grant to me purity of heart, so that I many honor You. For I have come to know that by honoring women and recognizing their creation in Your image, then I honor You, Father God. Thank you for saving me, God. Teach me to lead others.

In Jesus' Holy, Holy Name,

Amen.

If you could choose any man of the Bible, besides Jesus, to sit down a speak with, who would it be? For me, it would be Paul. But who is it for you? And what questions would you ask him? You can write them down here, if you'd like.

Share what you learned this week with your prayer partner this week. Let him know how you're progressing in your journey. And we'd love for you to contact us at www.jobswarriorsmensministry.com and let us know how things are going!

Open your eyes, Fantasy Seeker, for I am trapped in a nightmare while being forced to fulfill your dream. You compartmentalize this dark corner of your life as you step back out into the daylight while leaving me here... If only you could see that what pleases you is killing me. If I fail to perform and sell you what you seek... if I am not able to service you through my abuse and pain, there will be severe consequences. But you will never see them, because all you see is the sex fantasy. Open your eyes, Fantasy Seeker, because your satisfaction may be the death of me.

—Poem by Sula Skiles, Survivor of Human Trafficking

Lesson VII

Pornography

But I say, anyone who even looks at a woman
with lust has already committed adultery with her in his heart.
—Matthew 5:28

Pornography

The depiction of erotic behavior (as in pictures or writing) intended to cause sexual excitement; (2) material (as books or a photograph) that depicts erotic behavior and is intended to cause sexual excitement; (3) the depiction of acts in a sensational manner so as to arouse a quick intense emotional reaction.[3]

Yep. That's how *Merriam-Webster Dictionary Online* defines pornography. But I would guess that if you asked individuals on the street to define the term, you'd probably get any number of answers.

---

[3]   Merriam-Webster Dictionary online

Wikipedia does not stray far from *Merriam-Webster*, defining pornography as "the portrayal of sexual subject matter for the purpose of sexual arousal."[4]

The first reported image of porn in modern times was in the Victorian era, a time in British history that correlated with the reign of Queen Victoria from 1837 to 1901. Obviously, pornography in some form or fashion has been around much, much longer.

However, you might personally define the term pornography, it comes down to the fact that it involves glorifying the body of humanity, in particularly the body of woman, for the viewing pleasure of others. And it goes against all that God planned for male and female that He created in His image.

Although it doesn't meet the definition of pornography, and I am in no way suggesting that it does, the first mention of nudity comes during The Fall. In Genesis 3:7, it says, *"At that moment, their eyes were opened, and they suddenly felt shame at their nakedness. So they strung fig leaves together around their hips to cover themselves"*—the first record of humanity seeing nakedness. And because of what? Because of sin.

Look at where that has taken us. In our modern world you can find pornography anywhere. It has become a multibillion-dollar business. Interesting isn't it, what Satan can do with disobedience, with turning our individual backs on God? He took that one act of disobedience in that Garden, and now we see a multi-billion dollar industry that takes all that God designed and twists it to further separate man from God.

And look at what it has done to man himself. It has taken man, the male of the species, the one that God designed to lead His world of creation here on earth, the one whom God designed to honor and protect the female of the species whom was created in His own

---

[4]   https://en.wikipedia.org/wiki/Pornography

image. Sin has taught man to degrade the image of God in the most vile of ways. But then again, what should we expect of a species, designed and created to share in relationship with the God of the universe who then executed the very one who created him? I guess we should expect no less from such a thankless beings as us. It fits right in with the "what have you done for me lately" mindset that most of us have. I find it sad.

Let's take a look at some pornography statistics.[5]

- Porn sites get more visits per month than Netflix, Amazon, and Twitter combined.
- 30% of the Internet industry is pornography.
- Mobile porn was estimated to be at $2.8 billion as of 2015.
- The United States is the largest producer and exporter of hard core pornographic DVDs and web material, followed by Germany.
- A Google Trends analysis indicates that searches for "teen porn" have more than tripled between 2005 and 2013. Total searches for teen-related porn reached an estimated five hundred thousand in March 2013—one-third of total daily searches for pornographic websites.
- Of the 304 scenes analyzed, 88.2 percent contained physical aggression, principally spanking, gagging, and slapping, while 48.7 percent of scenes contained verbal aggression, primarily name-calling. Perpetrators of aggression were usually male, whereas targets of aggression were overwhelmingly female.
- A Google search for "bestiality" generated 2.7 million returns.

---

5   http://www.internetsafety101.org/Pornographystatistics.htm

- Youth who look at violent X-rated material are six times more likely to report forcing someone to do something sexual online or in-person versus youth not exposed to X-rated material.
- Middle-school aged boys who view X-rated content are almost three times more likely to report oral sex and sexual intercourse than boys who do not use sexually explicit material.
- A study in the southeastern U.S. found that 53 percent of boys and 28 percent of girls (ages 12–15) reported use of sexually explicit media. The Internet was the most popular forum for viewing.
- The words "sex" and "porn" rank fourth and sixth among the top ten most popular search terms.
- Roughly *two-thirds (67 percent)* of young men and *one-half (49 percent)* of young women agree that viewing pornography is acceptable.
- Nearly *9 out of 10 (87 percent)* young men and 1 out of 3 (31 percent) young women report using pornography.
- Internet pornography was blamed for a 20 percent increase in sexual attacks by children over three years.
- One out of three youth who viewed pornography, viewed the pornography intentionally.
- Seven out of ten youth have accidentally come across pornography online.
- Nearly 80 percent of unwanted exposure to pornography is taking place in the home (79 percent occurs in the home; 9 percent occurs at school; 7 percent other/unknown; 5 percent at a friend's home).

These numbers are astounding. But in your world, much like in my past world, you wonder, "what the heck does it hurt for me to look at a little porn?" But did you see those numbers?! How many men is that who are failing at what God put them on this earth to do? And look at the amount of *kids* who are viewing this stuff. Do you *really* think that is healthy for them? Now, do you see how important it is that you stop viewing porn and take seriously your role as a man in God's world? If we were all pursuing *God* instead of porn, think how much better the world would be.

Let's get our memory verse for this week at this point. This is an important one for you. Remember, you were created by God for a reason. Part of that reason is to be a man of God, a leader in some way that God wants you to be. Perhaps He has a higher calling for **you**, but that will only be found through obedience to Him and service to others.

Again, God created *you*, so your memory verse this week pertains to that:

[18] *Run away from sexual sin!*

[19] *You do not belong to yourself,* [20] *for God bought you with a high price. So you must honor God with your body* (1 Corinthians 6:18, 19–20).

If you choose to be a man of God, then the above words must become a guide for you. When we honor ourselves and others, we honor God. It doesn't mean we punish ourselves, it means we sacrifice to glorify God. If you stop and think about it, what do you think Jesus Christ did for you and for me? He was beaten and hung on a cross to take your sin upon Himself so that you might be saved and spend eternity with Him. So, isn't it only fair that you refrain from pornography, which leads to a host of other questionable choices?

Write this week's memory verse here:

_____

_____

_____

_____

_____

_____

_____

_____

Whether you realize it or not, or whether you agree or not, pornography is sexual sin. It is that simple. There is no other excuse, or explanation. Try as one might, it cannot be "explained away." Quite bluntly, it is not "okay," no matter what someone says to you. It doesn't matter whether you are married or single, gazing upon the naked bodies of others and fantasizing about sex with them or about them is sin.

Following are several biblical accounts of what sex is intended for, and how sexual sin occurs.

Do not covet your neighbor's wife (Exodus 20:17).

God wants you to be holy, so you should keep clear of sexual sin. Then each of you will control your body and live in holiness and honor—not in lustful passion as the pagans do, in their ignorance of God and His ways (1 Thessalonians 4:3–5).

Let there be no sexual immorality, impurity, or greed among you. Such sins have no place among God's people (Ephesians 5:3).

Can a man scoop fire into his lap and not be burned? Can he walk on hot coals and not blister his feet? So it is with the man who sleeps with another man's wife. He who embraces her will not go unpunished. But the man who commits adultery is an utter fool, for he destroys his own soul (Proverbs 6:27–29, 32).

113

The husband should not deprive his wife of sexual intimacy, which is her right as a married woman, nor should the wife deprive her husband. The wife gives authority over her body to her husband, and the husband also gives authority over his body to his wife. So do not deprive each other of sexual relations (1 Corinthians 7:3–4).

These are just a few scriptures that demand sexual purity of God's ultimate creation. Your leadership call as a man of God requires that you refrain from impurity.

Viewing pornography is not practicing purity; it is not refraining from impurity. Viewing pornography is not something that a man of God participates in, encourages, or tolerates. If a man of God is called to leadership, and to purity, then he cannot tolerate sexual immorality. He cannot tolerate pornography. And he must do all he can to lead people away from such activity.

Earlier you saw some statistics that showed the rampant of use of porn. Hopefully, that got your attention. If a man of God seeks purity, then the following statistics should concern you even more.

Child Pornography[6]

- Child pornography is a $3 billion industry.
- Child pornography is one of the fastest growing businesses online, and the content is becoming much worse (Internet Watch Foundation). Internet Watch Foundation confirmed 1,536 child abuse domains in 2008.

---

6   http://www.internetsafety101.org/Pornographystatistics.htm

- The fastest-growing demand in commercial websites for child abuse is for images depicting the worst type of abuse, including penetrative sexual activity involving children and adults and sadism or penetration by an animal. 58 percent of child sexual abuse images depict this level of abuse (IWF, 2008).

- 69 percent of all victims in child abuse images are between *the ages of 0 and 10 years old* (IWF, 2008).

- In a study of arrested child pornography possessors, 40 percent had both sexually victimized children and were in possession of child pornography. Of those arrested between 2000 and 2001, 83 percent had images involving children between the ages 6 and 12; 39 percent had images of children between ages 3 and 5; and 19% had images of infants and toddlers under age 3 (National Center for Missing & Exploited Children, Child Pornography Possessors Arrested in Internet-Related Crimes: Findings from the National Juvenile Online Victimization Study. 2005).

It is my hope that such statistics disgust you. If not, it is my hope that as your relationship with Christ grows, such statistics will come to disgust you. God addresses the way that children are to be treated. If you are going through this study having been a pornography viewer, and in particularly if that porn use has involved children, be aware that the following scriptures are going to be harsh. Remember, God expects you, as a leader in His creation, to provide, protect, honor. And those requirements go to your protection and nurturing of children as well as women.

But if anyone causes one of these little ones who trusts in Me to lose faith, it would be better for that person to be thrown into the sea with a large millstone tied around the neck (Matthew 18:6).

Beware that you don't despise a single one of these little ones. For I tell you that in heaven their angels are always in the presence of my heavenly Father (Matthew 18:10).

³Children are a gift from the Lord; they are a reward from Him. ⁴Children born to a young man are like sharp arrows in a warrior's hands (Psalm 127:3–4).

³Give fair judgment to the poor and the orphan; uphold the rights of the oppressed and the destitute. ⁴Rescue the poor and helpless; deliver them from the grasp of evil people (Psalm 82:3–4).

I'd say that God is pretty serious about how children are to be protected, and I'd say that children are very important to Him, especially since they can't protect themselves, and even less so than woman. Finally, I'd say that God is pretty serious about punishment that faces those who mistreat children. *"¹⁶Then Jesus called for the children and said to the disciples, 'Let the children come to me. Don't stop them! For the Kingdome of God belongs to such as these"* (Luke 18:16).

Yes, God is very serious about the children. To gaze upon a child in lust, in child pornography is indeed dangerous ground upon which to tread. If you are not concerned about the law of the land(s), you might want to be concerned about the law of the God of the universe. Do not mistreat His children. And while these last few sentences have been addressing little children, keep in mind that **all** people are God's children; and that includes men, women, boys, and girls.

It would be a wise choice to not concern yourself with pleasures here on earth, but to concern yourself with eternity. Life on earth, is, as James says, a vapor, or a fog— *"How do you know what your life will be like tomorrow? Your life is like the morning fog--it's here a little while, then it's gone* (James 4:14). Eternity is a long time. Sacrifices here are key to your eternity. Again, if Jesus cared enough to hang on a cross for you, dying an agonizing death, then how hard is it for you to give up a life of sin. And again, will you fall short from time to time? Yes. But with Christ, you can beat the earthly, or sinful, desire. Just remember, it ain't easy. Satan doesn't want you to win.

By the way, earlier, the topic of purity came up. You learned that viewing pornography is impure. Do you think that viewing child porn is somehow less impure? Based on the responsibility that you, as a man, have to provide leadership in God's creation, I'd suggest that dishonoring a child seems to bring even harsher penalties than viewing naked women (or men)!

If you are still a porn viewer going through this study, and you desire to be a man of God, you can see that changes absolutely must be made. No ifs, ands, or buts about it. Christ will transform you and will release the Holy Spirit within you, but you will face trials and temptations. God allows these trials and temptations to better shape you into the man He needs you to be. Think about it—would you run a marathon without first training? Would you expect to walk on to a college football team with no preparation? Would you expect to fix a car without knowing what you are doing? Would you want to go into combat without being familiar with the weapon that you are being assigned, especially if it's a weapon you've never before seen?

You *are* in warfare. When you follow the world, or evil, you don't feel the warfare, for Satan has you where he wants you to be— lost. Those little twinges of guilt or knowing that wrongdoing is occurring comes from the Holy Spirit; He is trying to get your attention. But God has laid out the game plan and He lets you decide which team to play on. He wants you on His team, but He lets you choose. Satan, on the other hand, wants you on his team. And he will do all he can do to get you there, and then to keep you there. If you decide to join God's team, Satan will do all he can to bring you back to his team, or he will harass you with temptation(s) to trip you up. You see, once you are truly transformed by Christ, then Satan has lost you. So he will do all he can to make your life miserable here on this earthly plain. You must study and pray (talk to and listen to God) daily, at least, to gain strength for the battles that the enemy throws at you. Just like training for anything. There will be setbacks, and there will be hard trials (training), but in the end, it is the training that lets you accomplish the goal and cross the finish line.

As the Apostle Paul says in 2 Timothy 4:7–8, as he neared the end of his own time here on the earthly plain,

"7I have fought the good fight, I have finished the course, I have kept the faith; 8in the future there is laid up for me the crown of righteousness, which the Lord, the righteous Judge, will award to me on that day; and not only to me, but also to all who have loved His appearing."

This should be a goal for you (and me), as you seek your place of leadership as a man of God.

In April of 2016, Denny Burk wrote an article in *Christianity Culture.*[7] The name of the article is *The Darkness of Porn and the Hope of the Gospel.* In this article, Burk found that, "a growing number of young men are convinced that their sexual responses have been sabotaged because their brains were virtually marinated in porn when they were adolescents. Their generation has consumed explicit content in quantities and varieties never before possible, on devices designed to deliver content swiftly and privately, all at an age when their brains

---

[7]   http://www.dennyburk.com/the-darkness-of-porn-and-the-hope-of-the-gospel/

were more plastic—more prone to permanent change—than in later life. These young men feel like unwitting guinea pigs in a largely unmonitored decade-long experiment in sexual conditioning."

While I don't totally disagree with Burk and believe that he has some good things to say about porn usage, I would argue here that it matters not about it being available on the internet. While it is true that pornography is more easily accessible than ever, men have always found ways to use women for their viewing pleasure. I can remember sitting upstairs in my home on the old desktop computer with dial up internet, seeing the same things one can now see. The only real concern with dial up was when you heard your wife coming up the stairs and trying to clear the screen before she got in the room. It was a race!

That being said, I do understand that internet porn is faster to get now than it was then. But I just don't think it's any easier to get. Even in the days of dial up, if you wanted to find it, you could find it. And even before the internet, if you wanted to find it, you could find it. I will concede that it is easier for those under 18 to access it now, and that it is surely a tragedy for our youth. I would agree that what a boy sees when he is young shapes who he is later, but I don't think it matters when he sees the image that brings that tendency to the forefront of the mind. Remember, I first saw images that stirred butterflies in my stomach when I was about eleven years old, but it was when I was twenty years old that I laid my eyes on the scenes in Penthouse that brought those fantasies to life.

The problem seems to be that for the pornography viewer, it becomes easier to view the porn than to try and be in an actual relationship. It somewhat became that way for me. When I was angry with Melinda, or felt powerless, I could always retreat to pornography and watch women do whatever I wanted them to do. I didn't have to communicate with them, for they were there at the push of a button, or the turn of a page. Burk says in his article that many young men "are simply unable to experience a sexual response with a real live woman. They are able only to respond to pornography. In fact, they prefer pornography."

Maybe this is you. Or maybe, like me, it was the porn that fuels your sex life with your wife. Maybe she is unaware of your thoughts when the two of you have sex. Maybe, in your mind, it is the only thing that seems to work to get you aroused for sex with her. Maybe you feel there is nothing that you can do about it.

Brother, let me assure you that Jesus Christ can handle it for you. He can take the desire to view porn, He can take the desire you have for fantasies, He can change the way you view your wife, and the way you view women in general. Jesus Christ truly is the way, the truth, and the life. He is your saving grace for your very soul in eternity, and he is the saving grace to pull you from the pits of hell in which you currently suffer in the world of pornography. Let Christ take it away. He can do it. And only He can do it. You cannot do it by yourself. You need Him. You need Him to teach you the purity, the leadership for which you were designed. Let Him have it. Become the man that you were created to be. Not a man of the world, or of evil. Not a man who dishonors women and children by viewing naked images of them or sexual images of them. I challenge you to become the man of God that you are intended to be.

_____

_____

Write your memory verse here:

Ending Prayer:

Heavenly Father,

I know longer want to be a man of the world. I want to be a man of God. Lord, I have had a problem with pornography for a long time. I no longer want to be that man. I no longer want to dishonor women (or children, if applicable) by viewing images of them nude or in sexual actions. I no longer want to dishonor You, God, by dishonoring them. Teach me, O God, to honor You and to honor them. Teach me to protect, provide, and respect them as Your children. Teach me Your ways O Lord, that I may live according to Your truth. Grant me purity of heart, that I may honor You.

In Christ's name,

Amen.

Wow. You may have learned some harsh realities in this lesson. What do you think? How did this lesson grab you? Kind of tough, isn't it? I'll bet you learned some things you didn't know. Write down what you're feeling, what you learned, etc. Write down what's on your heart and mind right now.

Now, when you journal, why don't you write all of this down in your journal? And you'll probably have some stuff to add. If not, that's okay. The Holy Spirit should really be prompting you right now. He is, even if you're not aware of it.

You may really have some heavy things to talk to your prayer partner about. Or maybe you just want to go to the Job's Warriors website and unload your feelings through our "contact us" method. Oh, it's all confidential.

Human Trafficking

⁸*Speak up for those who cannot speak for themselves;*
ensure justice for those who are perishing. ⁹ *Yes, speak up*
for the poor and helpless and see that they get justice.
—Proverbs 31:8–9

Human trafficking is the sale of a person, against their will, to another person for the use of sexual or labor services. In this lesson, you will be introduced to the various forms of trafficking. Human trafficking has been occurring since humanity, evicted from the Garden of Eden at The Fall, began to "be fruitful and multiply." I think you would agree that when God ordained population growth, He had no intent for this type of "commerce" to come into being.

Some who use pornography eventually graduate to the use of prostitutes. Many women in the porn images you view are not there by choice. Thus, pornography and human trafficking share a link. This link is not a good thing. In fact, it is a terrible thing.

If you are to be a man of God, a leader in His creation, then you must practice Proverbs 31:8–9. And this means standing strong in alliance with those who are used in pornography and human trafficking. It means fighting to end these two horrendous actions that are products of an evil world which fights against God's Kingdom.

Human Trafficking Statistics

- Human trafficking is a $32,000,000,000+ per year industry. It sits only behind drug trafficking in criminal enterprise.
- There are an estimated 27,000,000 people in modern-day slavery around the world.
- 800,000 people are trafficked across international borders every year. 50% are children, 80% are women and girls.
- 1,000,000 children are exploited by the international sex trade.
- 70% of female victims are trafficked into the sex trade. 30% into forced labor.

Domestic Minor Sex Trafficking in the United States

- There are 100,000 to 300,000 underage girls being sold for sex in America.
- The average age of entry into prostitution is 12–14 years old.
- 50,000 women and children are trafficked into the United States each year.
- 1 out of every 3 teens on the street will be lured toward prostitution within 48 hours of running away from home.
- Minor victims were sold an average of 10–15 times a day, 6 days a week.
- 1 out of 4 pornographic images is of a child.

- The sale of child pornography has become a $3 billion dollar industry.
- Over 100,000 websites offer child pornography.
- 55 percent of internet child pornography comes from the United States

Recently, I read in a study done by Julie Bindel called *Why Men Use Prostitutes*,[8] that "discovering the women were trafficked, pimped or otherwise coereced would appear not to be so effective. Almost half said they believed that most women in prostitution are victims of pimps ('the pimp does the psychological raping of the woman', explained one). But they still continued to visit them." More than half admitted that they either knew or believed that majority of women in prostitution were lured, tricked, or trafficked.

What?! *This* is what man has become?! The being that God created to take care of His creation, to protect the vulnerable, the woman, the child, has stooped to *this*? Is this who *you* want to be? Is this who you *are*?

It is my sincere hope that if you are going through this study, that you have either made a change in your life or are seeking to make a change in your life. Obviously, a relationship with Jesus Christ is most likely what brought you into this study.

After all you've done so far in this study, after becoming more of a man of God, I hope that this section, the previous lesson, and the one following are opening your eyes to see how important it is to man up and fight, as a man of God, these travesties that have damaged His creation. For me, to actually see that "men" know or suspect the women they use as prostitutes are trafficked is beyond explanation. *That is not manhood.* Yet I look at how man has been deceived by Satan, and I understand. I don't like it; but it is what it is. And

---

8   http://www.theguardian.com/society/2010/jan/15/why-men-use-prostitutes

that is the purpose of Job's Warriors; to empower men, through Jesus Christ, to stand tall and reclaim their manhood as God designed manhood to be; to stand tall and not allow women and children, whom God designed man to honor, respect, provide, and protect, to be snatched up by "industries" like pornography and human trafficking and used in an immoral way that goes against God's plan for humanity; to become the leaders of their own lives, their homes, their communities, their nations, and the globe that God designed man to be with the creation of Adam.

This is who *you*, the man going through this study, are called to be. Isn't it time that you stand up, cast off the desires of the world, and claim your role as a man of God?

It is my prayer that as you wind down this study, that you will realize your true potential as a man, and become the man you are meant to be.

Trafficking Avenues

Labor

- Agriculture
- Domestic Servitude
- Sweatshop Factories
- Service Industries
- Begging
- Child Soldiers
- Debt Bondage
- Organ Removal

While all of these types may not be in action in America, the truth is that those forms of labor trafficking do exist in other parts of the world. I find it disturbing that such forms can exist, but to me personally, it is organ removal that stands out strongly. If humanity is truly created in the very image of God, just who does one think he (or she) is to take the authority to remove organs from one individual to sell to another?! Come on, guys! Are you going to allow this?!

Sex

- Forced Prostitution
- Pornography
- Stripping
- Mail-Order Brides
- Live Sex Shows
- Sex Tourism

Wait? Pornography? But, but…

We'll get you more info on that in the following lesson. And yes, that stripper that's standing up there dancing on a pole just very well may not be doing it of her own free will. Chances are that anyone involved "for sale" in the sex industry either is not doing it of their own free choice, or at some point was a victim of human trafficking. They are now addicts because they were drugged, or used drugs or alcohol to deal with what they were being forced to do.

I want you to think about something. On page 79, there was a statistic that said victims (it's speaking of minors, but it's valid for adults as well) are sold ten to fifteen times a day, six days a week. Do you realize that if a person is subjected to a sexual act 10 times a day, that's sixty times a week? That's 3,120 times a year. Now, seriously, gentlemen—when is the last time that you had sex three thousand times in a year? Let's be blunt for a minute. The most I have had sex in one night, during my pre-salvation in Christ days, was four. Yes, that's four. And it was with someone I knew who was not a prostitute. Some of you can say you've done more than four in one night, some of you less. The point is, that after four I was spent and my partner was exhausted. Now, even in a highly active sex life, most people only have sex two to three times *a week*. That's 156 times a year. And it's consensual. Yet, there are people out there who are forced, against their will, to have sex over *three thousand* times in a year? And somebody else charges for their sexual services and keeps the money? Do you think that is right?! Do you think that is godly?!

And it's not just prostitution! It's pornography; it's stripping; it's "peep shows."

If you have participated in this as an "end-user," then you have contributed to the demise of another human being. Change that. Now. Let Jesus Christ teach you how.

Quite simply, sex outside of marriage is *not of God.* So certainly sex services are not of God!

Let there be no sexual immorality, impurity, or greed among you. Such sins have no place among God's people (Ephesians 5:3).

What the heck. Make that your memory verse for this week!

You know the drill. Write it here.

_____

_____

_____

_____

_____

_____

Excellent!

———————————————————————————

Over the last few years, significant headway has been made by states that have enacted laws pertaining to human trafficking. Polaris Project[9] has broken down those states into tiers, which shows the level of efforts made.

- Twenty-one states are tier 1, meaning they have passed significant laws to combat human trafficking.
- Sixteen states are tier 2, meaning they have passed numerous laws to combat human trafficking.
- Nine states are tier 3, meaning they have made nominal efforts to combat human trafficking.
- Four states are tier 4, meaning they have not made even minimal efforts to combat human trafficking.

According to these stats, thirty-seven of the fifty United States take human trafficking.

Seriously, while thirteen seem to be lagging behind in what is a huge problem in America. This means there are victims of human trafficking who are receiving little to no protection. However, the other problem is that those states who have enacted significant protections for human trafficking victims have only a few places to refer them to.

So I ask *you*, man of God. What do you intend to do about this? Now that you're called to lead, you can *no longer* sit idly by.

———————————————————————————

[9]   www.polarisproject.org

There are also tactics used by human traffickers to lure or trap people with low self-esteem into their traps (and remember, human trafficking is not only prostitution. It also includes pornography).

Tactics Used by traffickers

- Boyfriend complex: he sees a female who is lonely
- Social networks: looking for vulnerable males and females
- Drugging at social events: it happens, believe it or not
- Job opportunities: promises of false jobs that are actually trafficking traps
- Promise of things that you want: promises for the vulnerable or those with low self-esteem
- Sold by family members: yes, this does exist and is actually quite common
- Threats or coercion: threats against the victim or their family members
- Kidnapping: yes, some are literally abducted

All these tactics are driven by evil. They are in place to serve worldly (evil) men's desire for sex. And they are driven by worldly (evil) men's greed. If you are a man of God, you *cannot tolerate* this. For one man (or woman) to use others' bodies (lives) for their own profit is so ungodly that it's almost indescribable. You are in the beginning phases of learning who you are, and who God is. Do you want to go before God, when you die, without Jesus as your Savior? Do you want to go before God having not been forgiven of your transgressions. What do you think is going to happen to those who go before God with no sorrow or regrets for what they have done? More importantly, what do you think is going to happen to those who have no Savior?

Interesting, isn't it?

In addition to the tactics for luring or trapping people into becoming trafficking victims, the trafficker also has methods for "seasoning" the victim.

Methods of "Seasoning"

- Confinement: keeping contact with others to a minimum; often involves long periods of isolation
- Starvation: only feeding victims once or twice a day; often minimal food
- Physical/Psychological abuse: tied up, chained up. Told their family doesn't love them, etc.
- Rape/Gang rape: self-explanatory
- Beatings/Slapping/Whipping: self-explanatory
- Threats of violence against the victim and/or victim's family: threatening to harm or kill the victim or member of their family
- Forced drug use: using drugs to control the victim, causing them to become addicts.
- Burning: normally a punishment done by cigarette, lighter, or match
- Cutting: literally small cuts on the victim as a means of discipline
- Confiscation of legal documentation and identification: identification confiscated and "un-returnable" until the victim meets certain financial criteria which they will never be able to meet.
- Runaways: the trafficker will provide housing, food, beauty treatments, convince the victim that he is her boyfriend, then sell her body for his benefit financially, ensnaring her in a web of captivity.

As a man of God, you *cannot accept* this. It is your calling as a leader to fight these things. One human is not allowed to be subjected in forced servitude to another, for the other person's profit; not in your world as a leader in God's creation.

There are many other discussions that are necessary in the world of human trafficking, and if you want to join the fight against it, it is recommended that you find an anti-human trafficking ministry group and become further educated in this vial "commodity" and how you can fight it.

Quite honestly, as a leader in God's creation, you can't sit idly by while this atrocity continues to happen. You must take action.

Write your memory verse here:

_____

_____

_____

_____

_____

Ending Prayer
Holy Father,

I ask for Your guidance. I had no idea, or just refused to acknowledge, the problem of human trafficking. God, I realize that for people to be sold by other people goes against Your plan for humanity. Lead me, O Lord, in how I can best combat this atrocity of Your creation. Thank you, Father.

In the Holy Name of Jesus Christ,
Amen.

Uh-oh. This may have been another tough lesson, but wait. Why in the world in a Bible study to help me with my pornography sin is there a lesson on human trafficking? Well, read on. And learn.

Are you settling into a good church yet? How's things with your prayer partner going.

Hey. I've got a great idea! Why don't you go to www.jobswarriorsmensministry.com and share with us what you wrote in your journal yesterday? We'd love to see how things are progressing with you! Remember, we are praying for you *every day.*

Lesson IX

Pornography and Human Trafficking

Rescue the poor and helpless;
deliver them from the grasp of evil people.
—Psalm 82:4

Pornography and human trafficking go hand in hand. You can't have one without the other. While they could be independent of each other, the plain fact is that they are not. Many who you have leered at over the years in pornographic images are not there by their own will, nor are they there for your viewing pleasure. I used to like to think they enjoyed what they were doing, and that they were doing it for my pleasure. Guys, let's once again be blunt. The woman that you are gazing upon in a porn image, the one that you have masturbated to, chances are, gentlemen, that she is trafficked. Chances are that someone, often called a pimp, is forcing her to do this.

I'll never forget the disgust I felt, when I heard the story of a lady who said that she posed for pornographic pictures, and participated in pornographic movies because she knew that her pimp, standing there acting as if nothing was wrong, had a handgun tucked in the back waistband of his pants. She said that she knew she had only two choices—life or death. In other words, she knew she must participate, and look as if she was enjoying it, or that her pimp would shoot her and kill her.

Wow. Talk about a game changer. As I've said numerous times already, if you are, or are becoming, a man of God, then you simply cannot tolerate this. And let me ask you this and it has to do with the prostitution end of human trafficking—do you really think that people *choose* this line of work? **Warning**: Graphic comment following: How would *you* like to lay there and have a stranger ejaculate on or in you? What's that you say? Oh, silence. Yeah, I'm with you on that one. Is that what you think God created woman for? For you to ejaculate on or in her? Do you think that she is here only for your pleasure? Do you think that she is here for the pleasure of any other man that chooses to pay for her services? How about the woman or women in a pornographic image? Do you think they truly pose for your viewing pleasure? Do you truly think that they pose so that you can lie there and masturbate? Do you truly think that they sit there and think, "Hmm, I wonder who's masturbating to my pic right now?" I'm sorry; I didn't hear you. Oh yeah, I agree. I don't think they are doing that for any of those reasons—or having any of those thoughts—either.

How does that make you feel? Don't answer what you think people want to hear. Be honest with yourself.

_____

_____

_____

_____

_____

_____

_____

_____

_____

_____

_____

_____

_____

Yet often, in the male mind, deceived by Satan, that seems to be exactly what men want to think. That these people—women and children—pose with thoughts of men leering at their naked bodies or otherwise provocative poses. Nothing could be further from the truth.

Throughout this Bible study, you have heard that you are to _honor_ women. You have heard that by honoring women, you likewise honor God, because she is created in His image. You have read through different thoughts, reason, and biblical scripture to help drive this home to you, because we, as men—as humans—are by birthright selfish and sinful. There has now been scripture brought into the discussion that speaks of the poor and the oppressed. So let's ask this question; "do you really think that wealthy women choose to participate in pornography or prostitution?" Of course, the answer is no. Only the poor, the oppressed, the vulnerable, are most often targeted. And when you think about it, you could indeed call the vulnerable the poor or oppressed. Because it may not be that they are financially poor. It may be that they are poor in self-esteem, or poor in spirit, as Jesus often called it.

But I want to clear up just a bit more about honor and how lack of honor dishonors God.

Memory verse, and I hope that you are ready for this one. It's short, concise, and extremely clear:

*Those who oppress the poor insult their Maker, but those
who help the poor honor Him* (Proverbs 14:31)

Write it here:

_____

_____

_____

_____

There. Can it be any more clear? Can God have stated it any better? If you oppress, mistreat, abuse, take advantage of, use, prostitute, take pleasure in the poor, the destitute, the needy, the prostituted, the trafficked, the hurt, the chained, the beat down... then you insult, dishonor, mistreat, disrespect, hate the very God who made them. And, the very God who made *you.*

Will you commit to honor women? _____ Will you commit to turning your back on pornography?_____ If you are married, will commit to learning how to honor your wife? _____ (the blanks are provided for "yes" or "no." I certainly hope your answers are "yes." You will be provided a resource list to help you with these commitments at the end of this study.)

_____

Early on, it was said in the Introduction that God is indeed a God of love. A God who loves you so much that He gave His only Son so that you can have eternal life in His presence; a God that wishes that none should perish (2 Peter 3:9—read it).

But make no mistake. God is also a God of justice. And while He wishes that all will come to repentance and that none should perish, He will judge harshly those who mistreat His children; and in particularly—in addition to those who believe in His Son—the vulnerable, the poor, the oppressed, the needy. If you deny them, then you deny Him. *Is that what you want?* I hope not, brother. I hope not.

136

⁹And when the Lamb broke the fifth seal, I saw under the altar the souls of all who had been martyred for the word of God and for being faithful in their witness. ¹⁰They called loudly to the Lord and said, "O Sovereign Lord, holy and true, how long will it be before you judge the people who belong to this world for what they have done to us? When will you avenge our blood against these people?" ¹¹Then a white robe was given to each of them. And they were told to rest a little longer until the full number of their brothers and sisters—their fellow servants of Jesus—had been martyred (Revelation 6:9–11).

While this scripture pertains to the deaths of the actual followers of Christ, don't think that similar consequences won't exist for those who harm the poor, the oppressed, the vulnerable, the weak. Don't think that for a second. Any questions?

Need a few more words from God to drive it home? Okay. Here ya go!

Give fair judgment to the poor and the orphan; uphold the rights of the oppressed and the destitute (Psalm 82:3).

The Godly know the rights of the poor; the wicked don't care to know (Proverbs 29:7).

Learn to do good. Seek justice. Help the oppressed. Defend the orphan (Isaiah 1:17).

For I, the Lord, love justice (Isaiah 61:8).

O people, the Lord has already told you what is good, and this is what He requires: To do what is right, to love mercy, and to walk humbly with your God (Micah 6:8).

These are just more verses that make it clear what God expects of you as a man. Remember from lesson 1—protect, provide, respect, honor. You are to be a leader of God's creation.

It is vital that you understand that many of the women that you have been leering over in your pornography viewing are not there by choice. I know that was said earlier in this section, but you must see and understand the link between porn and human trafficking. And while it disturbs me that many, as stated earlier, seem not to care, it is my hope that becoming a man of God will make *you care.* I have also heard people be challenged with the question regarding the woman they are leering over as "what if it was your daughter?" Obviously, that doesn't seem to matter either. Guys, that is truly Satan at work. I am not calling you a Satanic man. I am saying that, without you even realizing it, Satan has taken you out of the game. He has taken you so far into the darkness that you are not even aware of your surroundings. I am hoping that as you have gone through this study, and as you read those scriptures above, that it makes you realize that you are in a struggle for the eternity of your very soul; and for the souls of others. It is my hope that you realize the lives that are destroyed due to the fact that Satan misleads the world, and pulls the world away from God.

This is not to make you feel guilt or shame. You already do, most likely. This is to lead you to the One who can free you, brother.

Continue on to find the hope that exists to free you from your sinful bondage.

[1]*And so, dear brothers, I plead with you to give your bodies to God. Let them be a living and holy sacrifice—the kind He will accept. When you think of what He has done for you, is this too much to ask?* [2]*Don't copy the behavior and customs of this world, but let God transform you into a new person by changing the way you think. Then*

you will know what God wants you to do, and you will know how good and pleasing and perfect His will really is (Romans 12:1–2).

"Open your eyes, Fantasy Seeker, for I am trapped in a nightmare while being forced to fulfill your dream. You compartmentalize this dark corner of your life as you step back out into the daylight while leaving me here... If only you could see that what pleases you is killing me. If I fail to perform and sell you what you seek... if I am not able to service you through my abuse and pain, there will be severe consequences. But you will never see them, because all you see is the sex fantasy. Open your eyes, Fantasy Seeker, because your satisfaction may be the death of me" (Sula Skiles).

Prior to this section on "Pornography and Human Trafficking," there was a poem shared that was written by Sula Skiles. It is shared here again. Then it is followed by further thoughts from Sula. It is my hope and my prayer, that as you step forward to become a man of God, that God will move you to tears through her words. And then it is my hope and my prayer that it will cause to rise within you an anger and a burning to desire to help people like her—men, women, boys, and girls—to be free from this life that they did not choose. And I hope and pray that it will cause a fire within you not to harm those who enslave, but to set them free as well, to help them find Christ so that they may have salvation.

This is used with Sula's permission. For more info, visit www. sulaskiles.com.

I remember the first time I heard the word "prostitute," along with other obscenities being screamed at me from a crowd of people. I was so confused as to how anyone could label me in that way when I was dying inside, being victimized by the sexual fantasy of another, and forced to give my body away to monsters. If only someone could have

*really seen me and identified what I was going through at the time...
not as a sex toy, or a sexual fantasy, not as a prostitute or a slut...
but as a victim who was screaming inside for someone to save me.*

*It's so easy to label and judge people while being completely clueless
of what is actually going on. I wish there were a way to shatter the
fantasy facade sold to customers of the sex industry while exposing
the dreadful reality of sex slavery. The eyes of the customers of
pornography and prostitution must be opened to the truth about sex
trafficking. As long as there is a high demand for purchased sexual
fantasies, there will always be some form of sexual exploitation.
The buying and selling of human beings for sex is a very lucrative
business. I feel compelled to, in some way, try to enlighten those
creating the demand (being a huge part of the root of the problem).*

*The illusion is extremely deceptive, leading many sex-industry thrill-
seekers to believe that the fun and sexy girl or boy in front of them
actually wants to be there to meet their sexual desires... that the money
used to purchase sex acts always benefits the one providing the services.
Wherever there is pornography or prostitution, there is absolutely sex
trafficking. I am not saying that all sex workers are victims. However,
more than likely at some point in their lives they were victimized
or exploited sexually in some way. With the average age a girl enters
the commercial sex trade being 12-14 years old and 11-13 for boys
(National Center for Missing and Exploited Children), I think it is
safe to say that everyone in the sex industry did **not** enter by choice.
I think prostituted people are extremely misunderstood, because the
dangerous consequences of allowing an individual to understand
could mean life or death. There is a **massive** difference in the way
someone labeled as a "prostitute" is perceived and the reality of what
is truly going on in their lives. So what is really happening in the life
of the individual trading or selling sex? Maybe most don't want to*

know the answer to this question. Maybe it's easier to look away and intentionally remain ignorant in order to continue satisfying the itch for acting out sexual fantasies. I am very aware that all customers are not ignorant to the atrocities and injustices feeding their addiction, but awareness may cause it to not be so easy to ignore or falsely justify.

The customer may see many things when it comes to engaging in pornography or physically purchasing a human for a 15-minute sexual encounter. The customer is being sold a fantasy of dolled-up bodies, appearing to want to do anything to please them sexually for a small fee... a knock on a truck door at a truck stop from a teenager seeking a sex partner may be all that someone sees... or a craigslist ad, in the "personal's section" listing a "new-to-town young girl, looking for a wild time" may spark someone's interest. Maybe a pornography collection seems harmless. However, there is another reality behind the invitation, the smile, the flirtation and all the right words being said to get customers to buy sex.

For a victim of trafficking there are different methods of force by puppeteers pulling the strings and controlling every move and action behind the scenes. Traffickers and pimps use physical violence, death threats of family members, forced drug addiction and dependence, emotional manipulation, verbal abuse, tricks and lies, debt bondage and other forms of manipulation. Behind the sexual fantasy that a customer enjoys in a cozy hotel room may be a kidnapped girl, beaten into submission, fighting withdrawals from a drug addiction forced on her, fearing for the lives of her family members, knowing that any day she could die if she fails to make the quota her pimp demands. But all you see is a fantasy... because her life depends on it.

I believe that awareness and prevention is powerful for all members of society. We can work together to put an end to this social injustice. The more that people are aware, the more likely they'll be able to identify victims of trafficking, and those who were once invisible won't be anymore. My hope is that consumers of pornography and customers of prostitution would continue being exposed to awareness, and that it would become less comfortable and more of a risk punishable by law to continue down the path they are on. Ultimately, customers can get help and find freedom, so they stop contributing to the demand for sex trafficking.

I am so thankful for all of the efforts of the anti-trafficking community and for organizations like Truckers Against Trafficking who work around the clock to make these dreams of abolishing modern-day slavery a reality. If we continue fighting in unity, the truth beyond the sex fantasy can be exposed, making a huge difference and freeing many.

Finally, to fight pornography and human trafficking,

⁹Don't just pretend that you love others. Really love them. Hate what is wrong. Stand on the side of the good. ¹⁰Love each other with genuine affection, and take delight in honoring each other (Romans 12:9–10).

Women do not belong in bondage. It is a man of God's calling to free them.

Write your memory verse

_____

_____

_____

_____

Ending Prayer
God,

Wow, Lord. I really had no clue as to the travesty of Your justice that I have committed. I had no idea that when I leered over images in pornography that those people may be the oppressed which You direct us to take care of. I realize that I have been not only abusing them, but spitting in the very face of Your Holy Word, Lord. Please forgive me. Please cleanse me, Lord, and show me the way out of the guilt and shame. I know that I am Yours; but I also now understand that they are Yours, too. Teach me, God, how to help myself first, so that I can then learn how to help others. Thank you for all You have done for me throughout life, even when I didn't realize or accept it. Make me Yours, God.

In the everlasting Name of Jesus Christ I ask these things,
Amen.

Ahhhh. Now you see why there was a lesson on human trafficking. I'll be honest, while I don't want you to feel guilt and shame (remember, Jesus handles that for you), I do hope you feel the same disgust I did when I learned that women were not posing "for me"; or "for you," for that matter. Most are posing because they are forced to. Honestly, that should make you feel sick for them. And now, instead of wanting to gaze upon them, it is my hope and prayer that you want to free them. This is a necessary time for fervent prayer, with and without your Prayer Partner. And, as much as you may ready to join the fight against porn and trafficking, trust me. You're not ready. You are still in a state of vulnerability, and Satan will use that. Don't yet go into the battle. It's going to take some time, maybe even a couple of years. Get strong first.

Lesson X

The Warrior Job

I made a covenant with my eyes never to look lustfully upon a woman.
—Job 31:1

The verse behind Job's Warriors: 31:1. The verse that is the inspiration for Job's Warriors Bible Study and ministry. The verse that says who we are, who I am, and hopefully, who you are becoming. Make it your memory verse for this lesson. Write it here:

_____

_____

_____

    To me, this verse is the strongest verse in God's Word to speak against pornography and against human trafficking. It says it all. These are the words that speak out and say, "I have become clean"! To avoid looking at a woman lustfully, is to make a vow. A strong vow. A vow in support of God and His creation of woman. A vow against pornography and human trafficking. Thus the name of this study—*Job's Warriors: Fighting to End Pornography and Human Trafficking*. Because if you are going to vow to help God's children, then you must stand strong against these sinful entities.

In all honesty, the verse above reads that the covenant was made not to look at a virgin, or young woman. And in all honesty, that is what you most often find in pornography and prostitution. Most men want to leer at, I mean, excuse me, view upon, young women or even girls. Not older women. But the gist behind Job's Warriors is to respect and honor *all* women, from birth to death.

Obviously, the verse that is the "trademark verse" for Job's Warriors is part of the reason that the name "Job's Warriors" was chosen. Yet, it was also because of who Job was. Job? Really? You're kidding, right? I mean, Job is often called the "Suffering Servant." And it is often also said that the book of Job teaches us to trust God, despite devastating tragedies that occur; that when it all falls apart, that trust in God is the most important thing.

But most importantly, regarding this verse, it was my own mantra, my own guideline, when I accepted Christ in 2011. I was first introduced to the verse in a book that I highly recommend and that will be listed in the resource section at the end of this study. It is called *Every Man's Battle*, written by Stephen Arterburn and Fred Stoeker. Jesus Christ transformed me, but He used the Every Man's series of books to effect the change that was necessary in my life. *Every Man's Battle, Every Man's Marriage, and Every Man God's Man* were crucial in my walk of faith in God.

In fact, in *Every Man's Battle*, Arterburn and Stoeker introduced me to this verse and to a concept called *bouncing your eyes*.[10] In this concept, I was taught to take notice when I was checking out a woman. Now, you must remember, that for me, it wasn't about just the fact that she was "hot," it was about taking a mental picture so later I could fantasize about her being with my wife. So while I was leering for the obvious reason, I also had deeper, darker thoughts

---

[10]   Arterburn, Stephen and Stoeker, Fred, *Every Man's Battle—Every Man's Guide to Winning the War on Sexual Temptation One Victory at a Time;* Waterbrook Press, Colorado Springs, CO, 2000.

going on. Chances are, that a good percentage of you reading right now face that same challenge. I really didn't realize just how much I did indeed notice other women. However, when I started *bouncing my eyes*, I found that I was looking a lot more than I realized! As part of the *bouncing your eyes* practice, when you notice yourself looking, you are to tell yourself that you have no authority to look at that; it doesn't belong to you. Wow. What a great concept; and it works. But it doesn't just work for people you see live and in person! It also works when you see pornography, or when you see images in magazines, television, on the internet, etc.! And *bouncing my eyes* was a key to my own healing.

Thus, part of the reason that Job's Warriors was born. Because of the profound effect that *bouncing my eyes* had on me! (Thanks, Fred and Stephen!) ☺

The other reason I chose to pattern this study after Job was because of his overwhelming strength. As said earlier, he is called the *Suffering Servant*. And he was an extremely humble man who did not show any traditional warrior traits. He wasn't a mighty warrior like Joshua, or a strong leader like Moses. He wasn't a great communicator like Paul, or a trail blazer like John the Baptist. No, he was more like you and me. A man who was not called by God to do some great feat, or to lead His people out of some strange land. He was kind of quiet; he was very humble. But when you read the story of Job, what you find is, in my opinion, one of the mightiest men in the Bible. He did indeed suffer lots more than most did, but he endured, he stayed strong, he kept his faith in Almighty God. And like you and me, he had a time where he questioned God and questioned his own worth. But he stayed the course, and he became a great man. He showed strength, resilience, and fortitude as he underwent tremendous struggles that most of us will never have to endure.

And that is why Job was chosen as the namesake for this Bible study and for this ministry; because it takes strength, resilience, and fortitude to turn away from pornography and to become the man that God calls you to be—leader, protector, provider. A man of honor who honors and respects women. A man of honor who honors and respects all. It takes a man of God to make a covenant with his eyes to never look lustfully upon a woman.

There are a lot of interesting things about Job, and about his story in God's Word. You can find it just prior to the Psalms. Most books of the Bible are known as to authorship, or at least some can be speculated to as to who wrote them. Not so with Job; in fact, it is not known who wrote Job. The date it was written is not even really known, but it's thought to have been written in the 1100s BC or earlier. And it's really about a man who had it all, lost it all, and was then restored. It's often said that the book of Job is about suffering and wisdom. This is true. But I'd dare add that it's also about faith, endurance, and restoration.

And isn't that what you need? Faith and endurance, surely. But mainly you need and seek restoration—salvation.

The book of Job shows that although God allowed "bad" things to happen to Job, it is Satan, not God, who is responsible for these "bad" things. Just like in your own life. As you seek freedom from the trap of pornography, it is not God, but Satan who has placed this in your life. God has simply allowed you to make a choice—to follow the world (evil, Satan) or to follow Him (peace, reward). And although God did allow Satan to taunt Job, it came down to choice. You see, Satan thought that if Job had all of his good taken away, then he would no longer love and trust God. He thought that if Job was given a *choice*, then he would no longer choose God; that he would turn his back on God. And God allowed this test, as He gives us free will. It's much like what you and I face every day. The world taunts, teases, and tempts us with those things which, in our minds, provide short-term pleasure. In fact, the decisions that you and I make based on our worldly desire (short-term pleasure) end up having long term effects on us and on those around us. Job chose wisely. What will you choose?

_____

_____

_____

_____

_____

_____

So who exactly was Job?

Job was basically a simple man. He was successful though, as he had attained wealth. Some, when they become successful, forget their roots. Job didn't. He remained faithful to God, acknowledging that it was God's blessings which allowed him his wealth. Take a look at how the book of Job starts, as stated in scripture.

Job's First Test

[6] One day the members of the heavenly court came to present themselves before the Lord, and the Accuser, Satan, came with them. [7] "Where have you come from?" the Lord asked Satan.

Satan answered the Lord, "I have been patrolling the earth, watching everything that's going on."

[8] Then the Lord asked Satan, "Have you noticed my servant Job? He is the finest man in all the earth. He is blameless—a man of complete integrity. He fears God and stays away from evil."

[9] Satan replied to the Lord, "Yes, but Job has good reason to fear God. [10] You have always put a wall of protection around him and his home and his property. You have made him prosper in

everything he does. Look how rich he is! [11] *But reach out and take away everything he has, and he will surely curse you to your face!"*

[12] *"All right, you may test him," the Lord said to Satan. "Do whatever you want with everything he possesses, but don't harm him physically." So Satan left the Lord's presence.*

The first thing that should be noticed is that God and Satan actually have a conversation. That's interesting in itself. Satan, who tried to overthrow God, still has access to God. But did you notice verse 12? Many seem not to know of this verse. Many blame God for their trials and tribulations; but it is made clear here that God *is not* responsible. While He allows it, it is not God who causes it! It is Satan. And due to our very sin nature that we have discussed throughout this study, we blame our Creator for wreaking havoc on us. Yet, He is the deliverer, not the havoc maker.

Once God gave Satan permission to test Job, Satan unleashed a series of calamities upon him; and they were severe. Read in your Bible Job 1:13–19.

Summarize here all that happened:

_____

_____

_____

_____

_____

_____

_____

_____

_____

_____

_____

_____

_____

_____

_____

_____

_____

_____

_____

_____

_____

Whew! That's a lot of stuff! And none of it good! How in the heck would *you* have reacted to all of this?! It's pretty devastating. First, an enemy stole all of his animals (a sign of wealth in Job's time), and killed all but one farmhand! Yet, as the one spoke, another arrived to tell Job that all of his sheep and shepherds had been killed! And then a third messenger comes in and advises Job that another enemy came upon his camels and servants and stole the camels and killed the servants! Whoa! All of this?! Yet, a fourth comes in and tells Job that a "powerful wind" (speculated to be a tornado) blew in, destroyed the house, and killed all of his sons and daughters! That's enough to drive anyone to despair!

Yet Job maintained his faith. Read verses 20–22. Write here those verses describing Job's response to all of this tragedy:

_____

_____

_____

_____

_____

_____

_____

_____

_____

_____

_____

_____

_____

After all that happened, Job remained faithful to God.

_____

_____

Job's Second Test

²*One day the members of the heavenly court came again to present themselves before the Lord, and the Accuser, Satan, came with them.* ² *"Where have you come from?" the Lord asked Satan.*

Satan answered the Lord, "I have been patrolling the earth, watching everything that's going on."

³ *Then the Lord asked Satan, "Have you noticed my servant Job? He is the finest man in all the earth. He is blameless—a man of complete integrity. He fears God and stays away from evil. And he has maintained his integrity, even though you urged me to harm him without cause."*

⁴ *Satan replied to the Lord, "Skin for skin! A man will give up everything he has to save his life.* ⁵ *But reach out and take away his health, and he will surely curse you to your face!"*

⁶ "All right, do with him as you please," the Lord said to Satan. "But spare his life."⁷ So Satan left the Lord's presence, and he struck Job with terrible boils from head to foot.

⁸ Job scraped his skin with a piece of broken pottery as he sat among the ashes. ⁹ His wife said to him, "Are you still trying to maintain your integrity? Curse God and die."

¹⁰ But Job replied, "You talk like a foolish woman. Should we accept only good things from the hand of God and never anything bad?" So in all this, Job said nothing wrong.

Wow. Covered from head to toe in boils, mocked by his wife, yet he continues to hold fast to his faith in God. If you've never had a boil, then you have no idea of the pain they inflict. I would occasionally get one when I was a kid. My dad, who was a doctor, would apply warm compresses to encourage the fluid to drain out. They were awful and painful sores. I probably had two in my lifetime, and they were when I was younger than ten years old. I can't imagine being covered over my entire body, as Job suffered. Yet, he remained strong. He remained resolved in his faith in God. When his wife questioned his resilience to God, he made it clear that both good and bad should be accepted. Would you agree (yes or no) that we tend to be faithful when things are good, yet we abandon God when things go wrong? _____

The remainder of the book of Job centers around these calamities that struck him, and it involves a series of discussions between Job and 3 of his friends, who attempt to give him "advice." Job does have despair and wonders where it all leads (have you done that?), but ultimately he knows that God is in control and that he is blessed by God despite all of the bad that has happened. But even as his friends suggest he shouldn't be so loyal, he remains faithful to God.

But it is in the first few verses of chapter 31 where the heart of Job's Warriors comes into play; it is these verses that give us the resolve we need to step forward and step up to honor, respect, and yes, to defend women. There are some verses that are in bold. Pay attention to those statements.

*31 **"I made a covenant with my eyes
not to look with lust at a young woman.***
*² For what has God above chosen for us?
What is our inheritance from the Almighty on high?
³ Isn't it calamity for the wicked
and misfortune for those who do evil?*
*⁴ **Doesn't He see everything I do
and every step I take?***
*⁵ "Have I lied to anyone
or deceived anyone?*
*⁶ Let God weigh me on the scales of justice,
for He knows my integrity.*
*⁷ If I have strayed from His pathway,
or if my heart has lusted for what my eyes have seen,
or if I am guilty of any other sin,*
*⁸ then let someone else eat the crops I have planted.
Let all that I have planted be uprooted.*
*⁹ "If my heart has been seduced by a woman,
or if I have lusted for my neighbor's wife,*
*¹⁰ then let my wife serve another man;
let other men sleep with her.*
*¹¹ **For lust is a shameful sin,
a crime that should be punished.***
*¹² It is a fire that burns all the way to hell.
It would wipe out everything I own.*

First of all, Job made a covenant with his eyes. You see above what that covenant was (verse 1).

God saw everything that Job did (verse 4). He sees all that I do; and, yes, He sees all that you do as well. You cannot hide from God. It is impossible (*Can anyone hide from me in a secret place? Am I not everywhere in all the heavens and earth?" says the LORD [Jeremiah 23:24]*).

God knew Job's integrity. He knows your integrity (or lack thereof—see Jeremiah 23:24 above, again, if necessary).

Job states that lust is a shameful sin; so much so that should he lust for another woman, that his crops be eaten by others and may other men sleep with his own wife. Guys, in Job's time, those two things are a big deal. First, it is not manly or respectful that your wife would sleep with other men; second, you often eat from your own crops, so for others to eat them renders you hungry. And whether or not you want to admit it, when you view pornography, you are lusting. When you look sexually at any woman besides your wife, you are lusting. It's that simple. Remember the memory verse from Matthew 5:28 in lesson 7? Write it here:

_____

_____

_____

_____

_____

_____

And lastly, it would wipe out everything that Job owns. And yes, it will wipe out everything that you own—physically, mentally, financially, and most importantly, spiritually. But you can change it all. You can become one of Job's Warriors, fighting for justice for those used by others.

154

By the way, in the end, due to his steadfastness, Job is restored by God, and he becomes even more blessed. And that can be your story, too. You may not receive bountiful financial blessings, but the eternal state of your soul can be salvaged, it can be restored. You can ensure where you will spend eternity. You can spend it in the very presence of God and have a fantastic eternity, or you can spend it with evil and out of the presence of God, miserable for all eternity. Once your time here on earth ends (i.e., when you die), it is too late. If you have lived a life denying Jesus Christ and living a worldly life with no thought as to how it affects you or others, it is over. You can't go before Christ in your eternal state and say, "Oh, wow. You're real. Well, you see, I meant to give my life to you, but, you know, I was busy." Nope. Once that time comes, it is too late. I have been accused in the past of trying to bring people to Jesus through fear. Truth often causes people to have fear. So it is not out of fear that I speak; it is out of love. I want you to turn your life around and spend eternity with me in the land of God!

Write your memory verse here:

_____

_____

_____

_____

_____

_____

Ending Prayer
Heavenly Father,

As I went through this lesson, it made it even more clear to me of the sins that I have committed in the area of pornography and lust. Cleanse me, O God, and give me the strength to turn my life around. When temptation rears its ugly head at me Lord, give me a way out.

God, I want to serve you, and I want to help those whom I used to victimize. Show me the way, O Lord; make me Yours.

In Christ's Name, I pray,

Amen.

Only one "directive" here. Job 31:1. Make the covenant with your eyes. Today. Write it down in your journal. And send us a message that you're making the covenant. God bless you, brother.

The Final Leg

Congratulations! You have reached the final lesson of this Bible study! Whoop, whoop! Great job!

This final lesson is different than the others. You have no memory verse this time (yes, I know you are celebrating that accomplishment)! And there are no "question and answers." It's straight stuff, baby!

And that's why it's called Finish Strong.

Lesson XI

Finish Strong

¹In the beginning was the Word,
and the Word was with God,
and the Word was God.
²He was with God in the beginning.
³All things were created through Him, and apart from Him not
one thing was created that has been created.
⁴Life was in Him,
and that life was the light of men.
⁵That light shines in the darkness,
yet the darkness did not overcome it.
—John 1:1–5

Sir, this is where it all comes together. This is where you begin to learn the responsibility placed upon you as a man, and, more importantly, as a man of God. This is where you learn your purpose, and why God created you.

This study has talked about several different factors in life. Its design is to free you, through Christ, from the use of pornography. It has shown you that those who pose for those photos probably don't do so by choice, and they certainly don't do so for your pleasure. It has shown that there is a direct link between pornography and human trafficking. It has shown you that these venues are not the product of God, but of Satan.

It has introduced you to both men and women of God. And it has talked about their shortcomings and failures as they sought to be men and women of God. It has talked about what the world (evil) wants you to be, and what the world (evil) wants women to be. And it has tried to point out that no matter what the world wants, it is your duty, your calling, as a man of God, created by God, to lead the world away from sin (evil) and to Christ; to lead people from darkness (Satan) to the light (Christ); to provide, protect, respect, and honor woman, who was also created from you, but by God. Thus, she, like you, is created in the image of God. Way back in lesson 3, you were shown the value of being created in God's image by sharing what God told Noah when he and his family left the ark.

All these men and women, like you, me, and everyone else here on this planet, are fallible. It shows that we all fall short of the glory of God (remember Romans 3:23—*"For all have sinned and all fall short of the glory of God [HCSB]*). We all fail, but we must continue to strive to be Christlike.

So now, you are introduced to the One Man who was infallible. The One Man who rose above it all because that is why He came to us. The One Man who, as God, took the form of the Son, and came to us. He came to us to do what we can't do for ourselves. He came to us, because His people were unable to follow the Law, so He came to fulfill the law, so that you, the man reading this, might have eternal life in glory with God, the Father.

Man of God, meet Jesus Christ. The Savior of the world, if the world so chooses to follow Him. The Savior of you, if you so choose to follow Him. Praise be to His name! Praise the Almighty! Sing praises to Him!

¹In the beginning was the Word,
and the Word was with God,
and the Word was God.
²He was with God in the beginning.
³All things were created through Him, and apart from Him not
one thing was created that has been created.
⁴Life was in Him,
and that life was the light of men.
⁵That light shines in the darkness,
yet the darkness did not overcome it.
—John 1:1–5 (HCSB)

It all makes sense. It just makes perfect sense.

If you travel back to the beginning of this study, back to lesson 1, you will see how this whole study started; much like the world we call home started. "*in the beginning.*" Look at the amazing similarities!

In the beginning, God created the heavens and the earth. The earth was formless and empty, and darkness covered the deep waters. And the Spirit of God was hovering over the surface of the waters. Then God said, "Let there be light, and there was light" (Genesis 1:1–3)

In the beginning was the Word, and the Word was with God, and the Word was God. He was with God in the beginning. All things were created through Him, and apart from Him not one thing was created that has been created. Life was in Him, and that life was the light of men. That light shines in the darkness, yet the darkness did not overcome it (John 1:1–5).

Do you see the similarities? *In the beginning* God created the heavens and the earth, and the Word was with God and the Word was God. *In the beginning* the earth was formless and empty and all things were created through Him and nothing was created apart from Him. *In the beginning* darkness covered the deep waters and the Spirit of God hovered above; God said for there to be light and there was light and that light shines in the darkness and the darkness does not overcome it. *Life was in Him, and that life was the light of men.*

Do you see it? Do you?

Jesus Christ *is* the Word. And Jesus was "with Him" during the very creation of the world. Jesus Christ is God and God is Jesus Christ. And the Spirit is God and God is the Spirit. Three in one. The Holy Trinity. Father, Son, Spirit.

Thus, when you deny Jesus, you deny God. When you deny the Spirit the opportunity to work within you, you deny God. For the Spirit is already there, you must release Him to work within you by accepting Jesus Christ, then by letting the Spirit guide you to follow Jesus Christ. *He gave His one and only Son, so that everyone who believes in Him will not perish but have eternal life* (John 3:16); *Jesus told him, "I am the way, the truth, and the life. No one can come to the Father except through me"* (John 14:6). Does it make more sense now than it did when you first started this study? *No one can come to the Father except through me.* Your primary calling *as a man* is to accept Jesus Christ as your Lord and Savior. As said *in the beginning* of this study, it is that simple. Yet, as you have learned, there are more things that you must do once you accept Him. You must become His disciple. You must step up. You must stand tall. You must stop viewing pornography, for to do so is to enable human trafficking and you are dishonoring women. And you must not tolerate God's ultimate creation being dishonored. For, as you have learned, to dishonor woman, is to dishonor God. And, *in the beginning*, Father, Son, and Spirit were present at that creation.

For when you let the Spirit work, when you follow Jesus, you follow God. *In the beginning.* Just like *in the beginning*, Jesus and the Spirit were present as God, and with God, *in the beginning* of your transformation in Christ, through that same Spirit, you are with God.

Jesus is your salvation in more ways than one. He is the answer to your eternity. And He is the answer to the trials and tribulations you will face when you come to Him. Yet, He never promised it will be easy. You have learned in this study that Satan is the bringer of all things bad; that he is out to separate you from God. Once you commit to Christ, Satan will do all he can to trip you up and turn you away. While it's much easier to just give in, don't make him happy. Stay the course. It will get easier over time. Jesus said,

"I have told you all this so that you may have peace in me. Here on earth you will have many trials and sorrows. But take heart, because I have overcome the world (John 16:33).

In all honesty, whether it's Satan, or whether it's just everyday life, Christ is there. Not everything is a Satanic attack, some days are just bad days. While bad things occur as a result of The Fall, it doesn't mean a bad day is a direct attack by the Evil One. Yet it is still a result of when darkness entered the world so long ago. Death occurs, and although death is a result of The Fall, it is not a direct Satanic attack. Sickness occurs, as does injury, sadness, depression, hatred, etc. And while each are a result of The Fall, they may not be a direct attack (though in some cases they are).

But no matter whether it is just a bad day as days go, or if it's a direct attack against you, Jesus is there. Take heart, He has overcome the world.

Perhaps Clayton King, a respected young pastor and founder of Crossroads Summer Camps, Crossroads Missions, and Clayton King ministries, says it best in his book *Stronger. Stronger* is a book that shares, as it says on the cover, *"How Hard Times Reveal God's Greatest Power."* King shares how God has brought him through tough times in his life, and how He has used different people at times to aid King on his journey. Because you see, when you accept Christ and become His follower, you begin a journey. There will be peaks and valleys in this journey, but if you lean on God as you move forward, you will learn great things and become a better and stronger man of God. King relates the following story, as he was dealing with the impending death of his sick father. He was taking his two young sons to the YMCA, trying to pull himself together before going in. I'll let King take it from here:

"The saving grace in all of this was that Jacob and Joseph were immersed in their movie in the backseat and were immune to the weight of sadness that had settled down hard on my shoulders. I didn't want my kids to see me like that. It would scare them. I swallowed hard and tried to pull it together, but it was hopeless. The grief was an unstoppable force. It was like trying to stop a freight train.

But I had to pull it together! I was driving the boys straight to basketball practice at the YMCA. As soon as I walked in, people would wonder what was wrong with me. Even worse, they would ask, and I would try to answer then fall all to pieces again, embarrassing myself and my kids. As we got closer to the gym, I prayed harder and harder for God to somehow, miraculously, give me the strength to get out of that car and walk into that building with my boys to basketball practice. But it wasn't working. I just kept crying. Ugly, uncontrollable crying.

We pulled into the parking lot. I would tell the boys to go in without me. I would sit in the car as long as it took me to compose myself. It was the weakest, most helpless feeling I'd ever known. As we parked, the boys took off their headphones. Then something truly wonderful happened. They immediately observed my frail state. I was broken and they knew it. Nowhere to go. No way to hide. I was unprotected and vulnerable in front of the two little boys that I'd been trying to be strong for.

Jacob spoke up. 'Joseph, Daddy is really upset. His heart is broken because his daddy is dying. Let's lay our hands on Daddy and pray for him like we prayed for Papa Joe, and let's ask God to give Daddy the strength he needs.' Then my children leaned forward. Jacob placed both hands on my left shoulder. Joseph placed both hands on my right shoulder. And they began to pray for me. Out loud."[11]

And there you have it. An example of a man of God, whose faith in God is strong, yet sometimes weak. He was vulnerable; he was heart-broken. Yet, he was trying to be strong. There is temptation in this state to "man-up" and handle it ourselves when we are in this type of state of mind. King could have done that, but he "manned up" the proper way that God wants us to "man up." He knew he couldn't handle it on his own, so he was asking God to help him. And God did. He responded in a way that I'm sure took King to a whole different level. I don't imagine that he ever expected his two young boys to respond in the way they did. But God uses who God chooses. And in this case He used two young children to comfort a man whom He claims as one of his own.

That's how God works. He uses us to get His Word out there, and He uses us to comfort one another as we journey through this walk that we call life. And just as it is your calling as a man of God to provide, protect, respect, and honor woman, you are not called to do it alone. You are called to do so as God directs.

But you can't learn this on your own. So you must learn from those who are already truly men of God. Through reading your Bible. Through prayer. Through fasting. Through church. Through reading books written by Bible believing men. Men who call on the name of Jesus Christ as their Savior.

Now, let's talk a little about who Jesus Christ is.

Jesus Christ is referred to as the Son of God, or the Son of Man. Jesus Christ *is* God, as shown in the opening scripture of this lesson. God is Father, Son, and Holy Spirit, known as the Triune God, or

11   King, Clayton, *Stronger-How Hard Times Reveal God's Greatest Power;* Baker Books, Grand Rapids, MI, 2015, 110–111

Holy Trinity—three in one. God created the world (Genesis) and created the Law for the Jewish population, His chosen people. Many people look at the Old Testament Law and mock it due to certain things that are written in the Law. What you need to understand about the Law is the complexity, yet the simplicity of it. If you follow the path of the Israelites (the Jewish people) after Abraham (remember him?) you will find a people who were offered everything for following God, yet couldn't hold up their end. This is what makes the Law so simple—simply follow God, and you follow the Law. For if they followed God, they would need no Law, for they would avoid sin. It is obvious from the history of the Israelites, as recorded in the Bible, that they failed miserably.

Enter Jesus. Jesus is often called God Incarnate, or God in human form. God is beyond sin; He cannot and does not sin, as He is all good. Jesus, in earthly form carried two major traits. He was fully human, yet fully divine. In other words, while still being God, He had human traits, therefore He could feel what we feel, experience what we experience. Satan saw Him as an easy target and tempted Him in the wilderness during his forty days and forty nights of prayer and fasting (Matthew 4, Luke 4). Yet, being God, He could face the feeling while overcoming. That is why Paul tells us to do our best to emulate Christ—overcome the feeling, the temptation.

Jesus also was the fulfillment of the Law. In other words, humanity was failing at following the Law, and only the Jewish people thought *they* could be saved by it. But just as the modern church tends to do today, salvation became about the Law, and not about God. In our modern churches, it often becomes about following creeds, traditions, or rituals; God is often forgotten. Jesus was the freedom from the Law, or today, from the creed or ritual driven church (Matthew 5:17—"*Don't misunderstand why I have come. I did not come to abolish the law of Moses or the writings of the prophets. No, I came to fulfill them*").

He overcame the Law by being the Law. Remember, as said above, if the Jewish people had followed God as He directed, there would be no need for the Law. Jesus says it best in Matthew 22:35-40,

[35]One of them, an expert in religious law, tried to trap Him with this question: [36]"Teacher, which is the most important commandment in the law of Moses?"

[37]Jesus replied, "you must love the Lord your God with all your heart, all your soul, and all your mind. [38]This is the first and greatest commandment. [39]A second is equally important: Love your neighbor as yourself. [40]All the other commandments and all the demands of the prophets are based on these two commandments.

Simplicity yet complexity. You see, if you'll follow these two commandments as a Christian, as a man of God, then you will follow *all* of God's Law, because you will have no need for Law. God is Law.

So when you gaze upon pornography, are you loving your neighbor as yourself? Or are you using your neighbor for your own selfish (sin nature) pleasure and gratification? Therefore, are you following God's Law, or the law of the world? Which choice do you think puts you in God's presence?

Jesus has also been called "the Second Adam." And that ties right in to the discussion above about the Law and Jesus' two greatest commandments. Just as Jesus came to fulfill the Law, He came to save humanity through grace as a result of Adam's failure. Adam was made *in the image* of God, yet was fully human. He could not hold up his end of the deal. Jesus was God in human form, and He was able to accomplish what Adam couldn't. Jesus restores. Jesus offers hope to a fallen world. He sets right what Adam caused. And He offers that to all. He offers that to *you*. Where you have been lost in a world of sin, of pornography, Jesus offers you the chance to come to Him and be saved. Saved from eternal damnation, saved from the life you now live, or have recently lived. And only He can deliver you. If you try without Christ, you will succeed for a while, only to fall back into the trap. If you go forward with Jesus, you will face temptations, but through Him, you can defeat the demon of pornography. You still may fall, but you now know the way out; and eventually the temptation is not as strong. A demon only spends time on you if he knows he can take you away from God. As he learns that you are truly of God, he will begin to turn his attention to easier prey. While he will come back at you from time to time, he will not try as hard, because he can't break through the protection that Jesus gives you, unless you let him. Eventually, he gets tired of messing with you, so he eases off.

There are other indicators, especially in the Gospel of John, that lead to this whole revelation that God is Father, Son, and Holy Spirit, in addition to the opening scripture in this lesson.

FATHER

[11]Just believe that I am in the Father and the Father is in me.
—John 15:11

SON

[21]Those who obey My commandments are the ones who love Me. And because they love Me, My Father will love them, and I will love them. And I will reveal myself to each one of them.
—John 15:21

HOLY SPIRIT

*²⁶But when the Father sends the Counselor as My Representative—
and by the Counselor I mean the Holy Spirit—He will teach you
everything and will remind you of everything I Myself have told you.*
—John 15:26

Father, Son, Holy Spirit. Three in one. Present at the creation, and present now. Offering Himself to *you*. Despite your sins, He beckons *you* to come to Him and be saved. *⁹The Lord isn't really being slow about His promise to return, as some people think.* **No, He is being patient for your sake.** *He does not want anyone to perish, so He is giving more time for everyone to repent* (2 Peter 3:9).

Repent. Be the man that God created you to be. Be a man of God. Step up and answer your calling to God. Do not continue to deny Him and the importance of His creation of woman. Provide for her. Protect her. Respect her. Honor her.

There are other interesting things about Jesus, but here is the wrap up. And if you don't know this, it's going to blow your mind. Remember the people we talked about in lessons 3 and 5 (you know, men and women of God)? Pay close attention. First, there was Abraham, the founder of the nation of Israel (as God promised him) was the father of Isaac, the father of Jacob (Israel), the one who didn't trust God and had a child with Hagar, his servant. That child, Ishmael was the founder of the Arabic nations which war with Israel to this very day. Abraham fell short, but was restored by God. How about Rahab? Do you remember her? She was the prostitute of Jericho who hid the Israelite spies and her (and her family) were saved from destruction by God. If you recall, she and her husband, an Israelite (Salmon), gave birth to Boaz (who married Ruth). From Boaz and Ruth came Obed, who fathered Jesse, who fathered David. Rahab fell short, but was restored by God. David, the King of Israel, who slept with Bathsheba, then had her husband killed in battle. A child was born of this illicit union, but the child did not survive. David married Bathsheba, and Soloman, future King of Israel, was born to them. Soloman built the Temple of God in Jerusalem. David fell short, but was restored by God.

Okay, so what is the point of all of this genealogy? Good question. You learned about those folks earlier. They all fell short, but God restored them.

Jesus Christ came from this line of sinners. Jesus Christ came from these people who fell short, but were restored. And then Jesus Christ died to save *you* from your own sins. If only you will let Him. If only you will say yes to Him.

God took the sin of man, and used it for His glory.

Final Prayer
Father God,

You have taken me on quite a journey as I have gone through this study. I have found out things about myself that I don't necessarily like. But I also realize now that the guilt and shame I have felt, and even feel today, come from the enemy and not from You. You stirred my heart by placing the original guilt upon me, but not that I am Yours, I know from where it comes. Lord, I have sinned. I have failed in my own efforts at life. Whether I have or have not been successful by the standards of the world, I realize that I have not been successful according to Your standard. Help me to right my ship, O God, and steer toward You and away from the influence of the world. Give me strength to resist the temptations that Satan will throw at me. Teach me to keep my eyes focused on You, and not on the world. Teach me how to help those whom I have abused, although at the time I had no clue that I was abusing them. Lord, I pray for cleansing from this life of pornography and sometimes even worse. I ask Your forgiveness.

Use me, O God, to advance Your kingdom and to introduce others to the salvation that You have granted to me.

Teach me to be a man of God.
In the Holy Name of Jesus Christ, Your Son and my Savior, I ask these things,
Amen.

Congratulations. You're done. You are free. Free in Jesus Christ. I praise and thank Almighty God for you. And thank you. Thank you for taking this step, and for stepping up to serve God and to honor women. You are the future of the sanity of this world, until the day that Jesus comes back for us. I am proud of you, I love you as a brother in Christ.

A Final Word

There has been a lot offered to you in this Bible study. A lot that I personally know will help you in defeating pornography. I have been where you are. While we may have walked different paths in the journey of sin, we are related. While all of us are related because we are created by God and because of The Fall, you and I are related in this particular leg of the journey. We both have been viewers of pornography, now seeking cleansing and freedom through Jesus Christ.

You have been challenged to learn the proper way to honor women, and leering at them naked and/or in provocative poses is not honoring them. But this also includes lust. That is why bouncing your eyes, so eloquently described by Arterburn and Stoeker becomes so important. For even staring at a woman in a way that you undress her with your eyes is also dishonorable.

But I do want to clear up just a couple of things for you. You are going to look. Everyone does. You will notice a beautiful woman when she walks in the room or crosses your path. And that's okay. Beauty, whether of a woman, or of another of God's creatures is just that—beauty. It's when you take that second look, or when you imagine what it would be like to be with her, or when your eyes divert from her eyes to her breasts, buttocks, or legs. At that point you are not looking at the beauty of one of God's creatures, you are looking at her as the world looks at her—as an object. And you are dishonoring her. You are dishonoring your wife. And you are dishonoring God. Save those looks for your wife. She is the one who deserves them.

As for honoring women, remember that just as there are men of the world, there are also women of the world. Don't become frustrated or down when they don't respond to your efforts as a man of God. People choose good or evil, salvation or damnation. All you can do is share what you have found—peace and salvation in Jesus Christ. Some will remain "in the world." You can't do anything about it. Your calling is to provide, protect, respect, and honor. If they refuse to accept it, there is nothing you can do about it.

In Matthew 28:19–20, Jesus commands us to go out and share the gospel (good news) with all of the world, and to teach His commands. And that's what you do now, as a man of God. You go and you share. If the world is unwilling to hear, you have done that part of your duty. Move forward in your own journey with God.

Lastly, find a Bible believing church. Attend and get involved. As you get comfortable with the people, you may feel led to share your story, much as I have done through this study. You may write something, you may be called to speak or to pastor, you may be led to share your story so others can benefit and become men of God.

I hope for you only easy times, but I know that will not happen. You will be tempted at every turn. So find someone in whom you can confide and whom you can talk to. Someone you can pray with. Get involved in other Bible studies to help you grow. At the end of this will be a suggested reading list. Many of these books were books that have helped me. If you can't afford them, check out your local library. If you still can't find them, contact us. We'll help you get one if we can.

Know that I am actively praying for you. I may not know your name personally, but if you have picked up this study, then I am praying for you in this battle. I ask you to also pray for me. It is easier for me right now, but I also know that Satan lurks at every corner, waiting for me to drop my guard; just as he will wait for an opportunity to pounce on you. We need each other's prayers, for the enemy cannot withstand the name of Jesus.

Know also that I love you as a brother in Christ. I and many others are pulling for you. And there are many women out there trapped in pornography and human trafficking that need you.

Journey on, my brother. Journey on. Stay in touch with God. And stay in touch with us at Job's Warriors. I hope that you go through all of the steps and become a leader in Job's Warriors.

Amen.

Bibliography

Arterburn, Stephen and Stoeker, Fred, *Every Man's Battle—Every Man's Guide to Winning the War on Sexual Temptation One Victory at a Time;* Waterbrook Press, Colorado Springs, CO, 2000.

Eldridge, John, *Wild at Heart,* Thomas Nelson Publishers, Nashville, TN, 2001, 2010.

King, Clayton, *Stronger: How Hard Times Reveal God's Greatest Power;* Baker Books, Grand Rapids, MI, 2015.

http://www.dennyburk.com/the-darkness-of-porn-and-the-hope-of-the-gospel/

https://en.wikipedia.org/wiki/Pornography

www.polarisproject.org

http://www.theguardian.com/society/2010/jan/15/why-men-use-prostitutes

http://www.internetsafety101.org/Pornographystatistics.htm

www.sulaskiles.com

Merriam-Webster Dictionary online

http://wordsfromwags.com/how-to-be-a-godly-man/

You have now completed a journey to free you from the slavery, the bondage of pornography. During this journey, you were introduced to Bible verses to commit to memory, verses that you can call on when facing temptation, but more-so to help you fulfill your calling as a man of God, a leader in your community, a provider and a protector to your wife, and ultimately to all women. Here again are the verses, compiled for you.

Memory Verses

Lesson I

Study this Book of Instruction continually. Meditate on it day and night so that you will be sure to obey everything written in it. Only then will you prosper and succeed in all you do (Joshua 1:8).

Lesson II

Teach me Your ways, O Lord, that I may live according to Your truths. Grant me purity of heart, that I may honor You (Psalm 86:11).

Lesson III

Keep asking, and it will be given to you. Keep searching, and you will find. Keep knocking, and the door will be opened to you. For everyone who asks receives, and the one who searches finds, and to the one who knocks, the door will be opened (Matthew 7:7–8).

Lesson IV

Above all else, guard your heart, for it affects everything you do (Proverbs 4:23).

Lesson V

Charm is deceptive, and beauty does not last; but a woman who fears the Lord is greatly praised (Proverbs 31:10).

Lesson VI

So my dear friends, flee from the worship of idols (1 Corinthians 10:14).

Lesson VII

Run away from sexual sin! You do not belong to yourself, for God bought you with a high price. So you must honor God with your body (1 Corinthians 6:18, 19–20).

Lesson VIII

Let there be no sexual immorality, impurity, or greed among you. Such sins have no place among God's people (Ephesians 5:3).

Lesson IX

*Those who oppress the poor insult their Maker, but those who help the poor **honor** Him* (Proverbs 14:31).

Lesson X

I made a covenant with my eyes never to look lustfully upon a woman (Job 31:1).

Ways to Get Closer to God and Become a Better Man of God

Find, attend, and get involved in a Bible believing, Bible preaching church

Read your Bible daily: Daily reading of the Word of God brings revelation to His Word for you.

Journal daily: Journaling gives you the opportunity to reflect on your time with God, including things revealed to you during reading of God's Word or just in interaction with people.

Pray daily (at least): Prayer is as vital as reading the Word. You don't need to have wonderful phrases to use during prayer; rather, just pray from the heart. Often, prayer includes quiet—rather than speaking, we listen for God.

Fast: Fasting is an opportunity to give complete control to God. Many people think that fasting means going for days without food. Not so. Fasting can mean giving up food for a half-day, or maybe giving up something you really like for a whole day, or for several days. Fasting needs to be done along with Bible study and prayer for the most effectiveness.

Memorize Bible verses: Hopefully you've already learned why memorization is so important.

Join a Christian Men's group: It is important that men build men in the faith.

Stay away from things, people, areas, etc., that tempt you.

If necessary, get counseling from a Christian, Bible believing counseling center.

Know that many of us are praying for and with you. You are not alone.

Recommended Reading

Every Man's Battle by Stephen Arterburn and Fred Stoeker
Every Man's Marriage by Stephen Arterburn and Fred Stoeker
Every Man, God's Man by Stephen Arterburn and Kenny Luck
Radical by David Platt
Radical Together by David Platt
Follow Me by David Platt
Not a Fan by Kyle Idleman
AHA by Kyle Idleman
The End of Me by Kyle Idleman
Stronger by Clayton King
The Prodigal God by Timothy Keller
Wild at Heart by John Eldridge
Walking With God by John Eldridge
The Radical Disciple by John Stott
Too Busy Not to Pray by Bill Hybels
The Bondage Breaker by Neal Anderson
The Christian Atheist by Craig Groeschel
A Man's Guide to the Spiritual Disciplines by Patrick Morley
Fasting for Spiritual Breakthrough by Elmer Towns
The Crucified Life by A. W. Tozer
In His Steps by Charles Sheldon
Five Minutes in the Bible for Men by Bob Barnes

Prayer: The Timeless Secret of High Impact Leaders by David Earley
Quiet Talks on Prayer by S. D. Gordon
The Good Book of Leadership by Borek, Lovett, Towns
Spiritual Warfare by Jerry Rankin

About the Author

Kevin is the executive director and founder of Job's Warriors Men's Ministry, a ministry designed to help men who struggle with viewing pornography. While involved with an anti-human trafficking ministry, Kevin was challenged by his wife to start a ministry that helps men who struggle with porn, due to the issues he had experienced as a porn viewer for all of his adult life until he found true salvation in Christ in 2011. It was obvious that porn has a profound link with human trafficking.

This started an eighteen-month journey of walking a path set by God that led to the founding of Job's Warriors and the writing of this Bible study. Kevin is ordained as a non-denominational pastor with Jesus Is The Only Way Ministries.

It is his hope and prayer that this study will help you escape the trap of pornography and obtain a closer walk with God. He can be reached at kevin@jobswarriors.org.